THE
HYPOCHONDRIAC'S HANDBOOK

THE **HYPOCHONDRIAC'S HANDBOOK**

SYNDROMES, DISEASES, AND AILMENTS THAT PROBABLY SHOULD HAVE **KILLED YOU BY NOW**

LANDAU, IAN

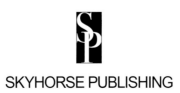

SKYHORSE PUBLISHING

Skyhorse Publishing books may be purchased in bulk at special discounts for sales promotion, corporate gifts, fund-raising, or educational purposes. Special editions can also be created to specifications. For details, contact the Special Sales Department, Skyhorse Publishing, 555 Eighth Avenue, Suite 903, New York, NY 10018 or info@skyhorsepublishing.com.

www.skyhorsepublishing.com

10 9 8 7 6 5 4 3 2 1

Library of Congress Cataloging-in-Publication Data

Landau, Ian.
 The hypochondriac's handbook : 33 Things That Probably Should Have Killed You By Now / Ian Landau.
    p. cm.
 ISBN 978-1-60239-970-9
 1. Hypochondria—Humor. 2. Diseases—Humor. I. Title.
 PN6231.H96L36 2010
 818'.602—dc22
                        2010004318

Printed in China

CONTENTS

INTRODUCTION

The opinions of my friends and family aside, I am not a hypochondriac. I do not wallow in worry. When I actually believe I suffer symptoms of various illnesses, my inner physician can diagnose—and luckily—treat them.

Still, I'm not a doctor. I can sign a prescription just like a doctor, but since I can't technically prescribe anything, my scribble doesn't mean much. That said, in the age of Internet research, you don't need a degree to figure out what's wrong with you. With this book, in fact, you just need the ability to read.

While researching, I was continually shocked by how many things can go so awry in the human body. From genetic mutations to infectious diseases, there are gazillions of ways our bodies—and our minds—become completely screwed up. Frankly, it's a wonder we've survived for as long as we have.

The twenty-first century has brought us major outbreaks of mad cow disease, swine flu, avian flu, and E. coli—and those are just the diseases you've heard of! What you don't know really can kill you, which is why I wrote this book. Start turning the pages, and you'll find a host of little known conditions and syndromes so horrible that your inner alarm bells will sound like never before.

But try not to freak out with anxiety (it causes migraines and ulcers). I've included ways to treat these problems (when treatable—some might simply kill). I hope at the very least you'll learn something new and expand the number of ailments you can draw upon when you can't help but feel "not right."

And now, I have to go, because my hand keeps doing funny things, and it just might be alien hand syndrome . . .

Ian Landau
2010

THE
HYPOCHONDRIAC'S
HANDBOOK

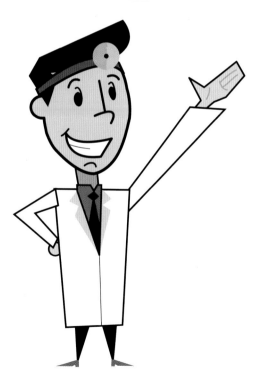

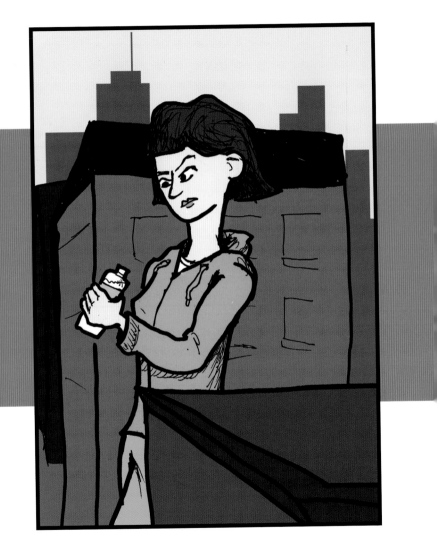

ALICE IN WONDERLAND SYNDROME

You're standing on a street corner, waiting for the light to change so you can cross. You've left work early because your head is killing you. "Goddamn migraine!" you think, as you absent-mindedly hum along to the soothing classical tune playing in your earphones (anything to shut out the grinding noise of the city).

You notice the "Walk" signal illuminate and prepare to step off the curb into the crosswalk. But as you take that first step, the weirdest thing happens: all of a sudden the other side of the street looks impossibly far away. And the crosswalk no longer looks flat, but is a series of undulating curves stretching to infinity, like waves on the ocean. You stop in your tracks and look around at the other pedestrians to see if anyone else is having the same experience, but that only brings on the next freaky phenomenon: everyone around you looks miniature, as if you're a giant and you might crush these tiny creatures if you take a step.

While you're still frozen in the road, the light has changed again and traffic is heading toward you. But just like with the people on foot, the vehicles coming at you look tiny, like little Matchbox cars hurtling along a child's toy race-track. The next thing you know, you're falling to the ground and then the world goes black.

When you come to, you're on the sidewalk and there's a crowd of people around looking scared and relieved at the same time. "That guy saved you!" someone says, pointing at a gentleman in a suit. But the main thing you notice is that everyone looks normal size again. You get up, assure everyone you're fine, and continue on your way.

Despite appearances, you're not crazy. The incident above could easily occur to someone suffering from Alice in Wonderland syndrome.

WHAT IS IT?

Alice in Wonderland syndrome (or AIWS) is a neurological disorder characterized by hallucinations and distorted perceptions of time, space, and body size.

ORIGINS

AIWS was first described in 1952 by C. W. Lippman in the *Journal of Nervous and Mental Disease*. It was named in 1955 by the English psychiatrist John Todd in an article for the *Canadian Medical Association Journal*, and to this day it is also sometimes referred to as Todd's syndrome. But Todd himself named the condition after Lewis Carroll's famed 1865 story, *Alice's Adventures in Wonderland*, and it's far better known by the name Todd gave it.

WHAT CAUSES IT?

The most common cause of AIWS is migraines (as it was in our sample case, above). It is well known that hallucinations are a common side effect of migraine auras (auras are usually associated with the onset of a migraine, and feature such things as zigzags of light, vision loss, and twinkling spots of light). Many doctors believe AIWS is a particular "brand" of migraine aura. Indeed, *Alice in Wonderland* author Lewis Carroll was known to suffer migraines, and many have speculated Carroll's inspiration for the tale stemmed from hallucinatory experiences during his migraine auras.

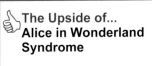

The Upside of...
Alice in Wonderland Syndrome

- Get acid-trip-like experiences without taking any drugs.
- The only upside of migraines.
- Adopt Jefferson Airplane's "White Rabbit" as your theme song.

Other known causes include epilepsy, acute fever, schizophrenia, Epstein-Barr viral infection, and infectious mononucleosis. A non-medical cause of AIWS is taking hallucinogenic drugs like LSD.

SIGNS AND SYMPTOMS

People suffering from AIWS may experience micropsia (objects appearing smaller than they really are) or macropsia (objects appearing larger than they really are), as well as the perception that time has slowed or sped up.

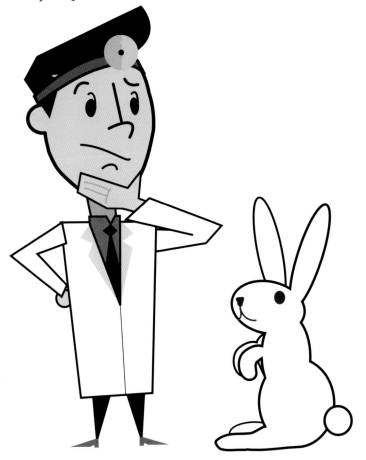

DIAGNOSIS AND TREATMENT

A diagnosis of AIWS is only made after ruling out other possible neurological problems or brain injuries.

Because migraines are the most common cause of AIWS, treatment is usually focused on controlling migraines through medication, diet, and adequate rest.

PROGNOSIS

People with AIWS have had mixed results in controlling their symptoms.

PREVALENCE

No statistics are available as to the number of AIWS cases.

HOW TO AVOID IT

The best way to prevent AIWS is to treat the migraines that appear to cause it.

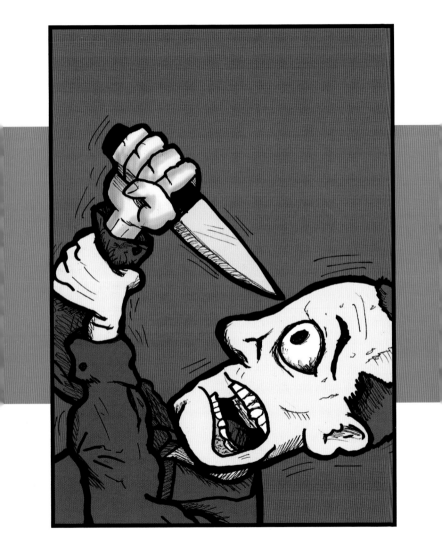

ALIEN HAND SYNDROME

You're sitting calmly, perched on your favorite easy chair, reading the Sunday paper. Your faithful dog is curled up next to the fireplace and Tchaikovsky plays on the stereo. All is peaceful and well in your world. That is, until someone starts pulling your hair. No one else was in the room with you when you last checked, and you never heard anyone enter. This is very, very odd, to say the least. You put down the paper and glance to your right, where you spy your right elbow at about shoulder height. Tracing your arm further up, it's all too clear what's pulling your hair: your own damn hand! *What the?!?!* You know you're not consciously pulling your hair; even weirder, though, you can't seem to let go! It's as if your hand isn't under your control anymore. Finally, you reach up with the left hand, grab your right wrist, and pull until you detach the right hand from your follicles. You rest your right arm across your lap and stare unbelievingly, unknowingly, at your right hand. Welcome to the wild world of alien hand syndrome (AHS).

WHAT IS IT?

Alien hand syndrome (AHS) is a rare neurological disorder in which patients seem to lose control of the movement of one of their hands. Feeling isn't lost in the hand, but many say the affected hand feels separate from them, or not a part of their body anymore. Unlike several other conditions that result in uncontrollable limbs, the hand movement in AHS is not a random tic or spasm. The hand moves purposefully and with control; it's just that the person whose body it's attached to has no control over what it's doing.

ORIGINS

Also called anarchic hand and Dr. Strangelove syndrome—after the famed Peter Sellers character in Stanley Kubrick's classic 1964 film—alien hand syndrome was first documented in 1909 by German neurologist Dr. Kurt Goldstein. Goldstein wrote of a fifty-seven-year-old female patient who claimed her left hand was "possessed." Her hand had tried to choke her, she said, and it had a tendency to grab her bed sheets and fling them to the floor. But it wasn't until 1972 that the term "alien hand syndrome" was actually coined by two French neurologists, S. Brion and C. P. Jedynak.

Since its discovery early in the last century, only several dozen cases of alien hand syndrome have been identified.

WHAT CAUSES IT?

AHS is brought on by damage to the brain's *corpus callosum*, a group of neurons that connect the left and right hemispheres. Damage to the corpus callosum may come from trauma, a stroke, lesions, an aneurysm, a brain infection, or hemorrhages, as well as being a side effect of brain surgery. Damage to these nerves scrambles communication between the two sides of the brain, and each side acts independently of the other. Thus you can end up with one hand that you have perfect control over and another that has a mind of its own.

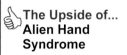

**The Upside of...
Alien Hand
Syndrome**

- "I didn't mean to grab your ass! That was my alien hand! No, really."
- Play chess against yourself—normal hand vs. alien hand.
- Call yourself Dr. Strangelove.

While damage to the corpus callosum is the major cause, damage to the frontal lobe can also bring on AHS. Interestingly, when the corpus callosum is affected a patient's non-dominant hand usually becomes the alien hand, whereas when the damage is to the brain's frontal lobe, the dominant hand is usually the one affected.

SIGNS AND SYMPTOMS

The basic symptom of AHS is involuntary movement of one of the hands. But just how that involuntary movement manifests itself can be pretty weird. Of course there's the joking example from above. In one case, a patient's anarchic left hand would constantly try to change the channel of the TV. Some AHS patients speak to their alien hand, apparently trying to reason with it as a way to keep it under control. One patient had a frustrating time playing checkers: his left hand would make moves he did not want to make, and when he moved the checker where he intended to with his right, the left hand would move it back. In another case, a woman's left hand tried to stop her right hand from holding a cigarette when she was smoking.

DIAGNOSIS AND TREATMENT

AHS may be diagnosed after brain scans and through talking with the patient about his or her case history.

There are no formal cures for AHS, but some treatment strategies do seem to help. Some patients have found relief by keeping the alien hand occupied, such as by holding an object in its grasp. For instance, one patient found that if he carried a cane in his anarchic hand, the hand wouldn't reach out to grab other objects. Other patients have covered their unruly hand with an oven mitt, and some have gone so far as to tie the hand up to stop it from doing whatever it wanted.

PROGNOSIS

There is no cure for AHS.

PREVALENCE

There have been roughly forty to fifty documented cases of AHS since it was first recognized in 1909.

HOW TO AVOID IT

There's little you can do to prevent getting AHS.

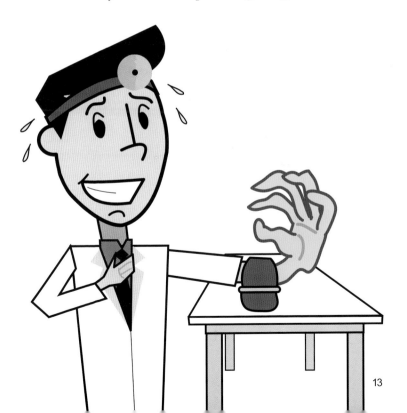

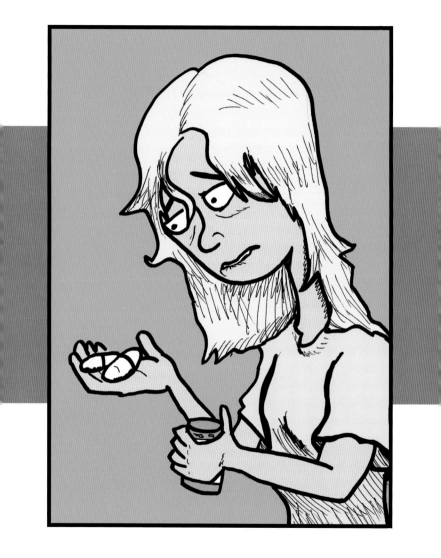

ANTIBIOTIC RESISTANT INFECTIONS

You're feeling sick—got a cough, a chest cold, whatever. What do you do? You call the doctor. The doctor looks you over and says, "Well, it's probably just a virus, but I'll give you some antibiotics just in case." Sure, couldn't hurt to zap whatever is ailing you with some good old fashioned medicine, right? Wrong! Antibiotics will do absolutely nothing to help cure a viral infection, like most colds, coughs, and even the flu. Antibiotics only work when you have a bacterial infection. And overuse of antibiotics—i.e., taking them when you don't have to—could wind up killing you! You see, each time you take an antibiotic unnecessarily, you increase the chance that it won't work when you get an actual bacterial infection.

WHAT IS IT?

Antibiotic resistance—aka, antibacterial resistance or antimicrobial resistance—occurs when illness-causing bacteria survive and multiply despite being exposed to antibiotic drugs. In a relatively short amount of time, antibacterial resistance has gone from being a minor problem to a serious world health crisis.

There are several different varieties of drug resistant bacteria, including: methicillin-resistant *Staphylococcus aureus* (MRSA), *Streptococcus pneumoniae*, vancomycin-resistant enterococci, multi-resistant salmonellae, and multi-resistant *Mycobacterium tuberculosis*.

ORIGINS

Since 1928, when Scottish biologist Sir Alexander Fleming first experimented with the antibacterial properties of mold, thus discovering penicillin, antibiotics have been a wonder drug. Penicillin, and the more than 150 antibiotics that followed it, have shortened illnesses and extended life expectancy throughout the globe. But

The Upside of... Antibiotic Resistant Infections

- "Hey, keep your coccus away from me!"
- Gives new meaning to the saying, "Resistance is futile."
- Make like Donald Trump—skip shaking hands.

the positive effects of antibiotics are increasingly under attack, as misuse of the drugs has dulled their efficacy, leading to drug-resistant strains of disease.

WHAT CAUSES IT?

It's quite simple, really. Bacteria are tiny, single-cell living organisms that can cause disease when they enter the body. (There are also "good," non-disease-causing bacteria that you actually want inside your body, such as those found in yogurt.) When you have a bacterial infection and you take an antibiotic, the drug targets and kills the bacteria that are making you ill, thus helping your immune system rid the body of the evil invaders. When the process works, you get better much faster than if you hadn't taken antibiotics, and your illness is often much less severe.

However, bacteria are tricky little devils, and every once in a while one of them has the ability to escape or neutralize the antibiotic meant to attack it. Some bacteria are naturally resistant to certain medications while others develop such capabilities, either through a genetic mutation or by acquiring the resistance from another related bacterium. And in the world of bacteria, the old Nietzschean saying, "Whatever doesn't kill you makes you stronger," certainly holds true. So now you have an antimicrobial resistant strain of some noxious bacteria floating around. That bacteria is then passed among people—through sneezing, touching door handles, shaking hands, traveling in an airplane, etc.—and pretty soon you have a bacterial infection that doesn't respond to antibiotics.

SIGNS AND SYMPTOMS

The specific symptoms of antibacterial resistance depend on what kind of bacterium has infected you. But suffice it to say, the number one symptom is that you simply won't get any better, despite taking your medicine.

DIAGNOSIS AND TREATMENT

How a drug-resistant bacterial infection is treated will depend on what kind of infection it is. Often when cheap, first-line antibiotics don't do the job, doctors will move on to second- and third-line medications. These subsequent drugs are typically much more expensive and toxic. Thus, you are sicker for longer, and the cost of treating you skyrockets.

PROGNOSIS

If detected early and treated correctly with replacement medications, many bacterial resistant strains can be killed off. If left untreated, however, these strains can kill you.

PREVALENCE

There are no exact figures of how many people are sickened and killed each year as a result of antibiotic resistance. But it's safe to say that the numbers are on the rise. A study of

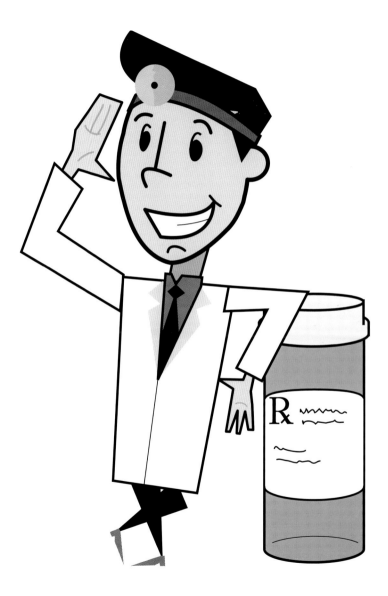

MRSA infections by the Centers for Disease Control and Prevention estimated there were 94,360 cases of MRSA in the U.S. in 2005, with 18,650 cases resulting in death (i.e., more fatalities from bacterial resistance than those caused by AIDS). In 2001, the CDC estimated the total number of MRSA cases at 31,440.

HOW TO AVOID IT

Be very cautious about taking antibiotics. Consult with your doctor about whether you really need to be taking an antibiotic for what's ailing you, and if you are prescribed one, follow the dosing instructions carefully. And for God's sake, wash your hands—often!

Incidentally, the world should probably be looking to Norway for guidance on how to handle the problem of antibiotic resistance. Norway is the most infection-free country in the world, a status it acquired over the past several years by drastically cutting back on the use of anti-biotics. A judicious program of prescribing antibiotics has meant that people don't develop resistance to them.

NOTABLE CASES

▪ Oswaldo Juarez

In the fall of 2007, a 19-year-old Peruvian man who'd come to Florida to study English went to doctors complaining of a severe chest cold. The man, Oswaldo Juarez, told doctors that his chest was tight and that he had an incessant hacking cough. What's more, he had started to cough up blood. Doctors discovered that Juarez was the first person in the U.S. to have a highly contagious, drug-resistant form of tuberculosis, referred to as XXDR TB. This form of TB is so rare that only a few people worldwide have ever been diagnosed with it. Stumped as to how to cure it, doctors treated Juarez for three months at a Fort Lauderdale hospital. But by December 2007, he wasn't cured and was subsequently moved to A.G. Holley State Hospital in Lantana, Fl., the last remaining TB sanitarium in the U.S. Juarez remained at the hospital for 19 months, while doctors experimented on him with different drugs. Finally, in July 2009, he was well enough to leave the hospital. His care had cost Florida taxpayers $500,000.

- **Athletes**

Proving that no one is immune to antibiotic resistant infections, some of the country's top athletes have been sidelined by an MRSA infection. Veterans like Grant Hill of the Phoenix Suns and Junior Seau of the New England Patriots have been struck, as well as West Virginia college basketball star Mike Gansey. MRSA outbreaks also have occurred at health clubs in recent years, pointing further to the seriousness of antibiotic resistance and the urgency to tackle the problem.

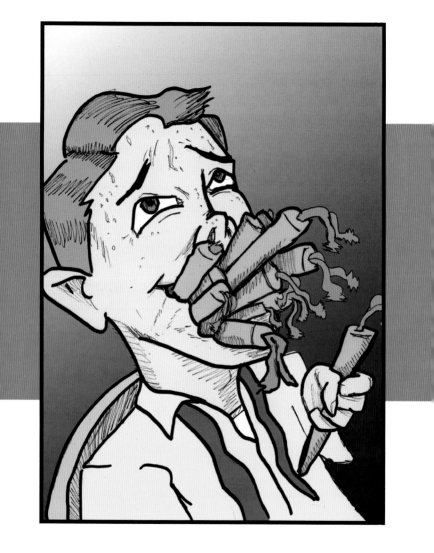

CARROT ADDICTION

What could be more harmless than a carrot? You've heard all your life about the benefits of eating these amazing root vegetables—"Eat your carrots and you'll have good eyesight," your mom said over and over. And if Mom's advice isn't convincing, there's always science: researchers say eating carrots does everything from preventing cancer to keeping your lungs healthy. One cup of raw carrots contains just 52 calories, but is loaded with vitamin A, not to mention vitamin C and potassium. Kids love 'em! Bugs Bunny loves 'em! But when it comes to carrots, love is just fine, and obsession is another matter.

It may sound absurd, but carrot addiction is all too real. In a 1992 article in the *British Journal of Addiction* entitled "Can carrots be addictive? An extraordinary form of drug dependence," Czech researchers Ludek and Karel Cerny detailed their view that carrots can be as addictive as cigarettes.

WHAT IS IT?

Carrot addicts consume huge amounts of carrots a day. And that doesn't mean absentmindedly munching through an entire bag of baby carrots while watching TV. Addicts have been known to eat up to ten pounds of their fave veggie a day. They can't help it. The craving *must* be satisfied.

ORIGINS

While carrot addiction hasn't been studied extensively, it has at least been known about since the early 1900s.

WHAT CAUSES IT?

There is debate in the scientific and medical communities as to the actual causes of carrot addiction. Certainly carrot addicts have a psychological dependence on the vegetable, but researchers such as the Cernys speculate that there is a chemical dependence at work as well. So far, however, no researcher has identified any substance in carrots that is known to be addictive—although one suspected culprit is carotene. In their paper the Cernys discuss intense withdrawal symptoms in patients who try to kick their carrot habit, thus lending some credence to the idea that addicts are more than just psychologically dependent.

Several of the case studies feature patients who took up eating carrots while quitting smoking. A number of female patients became addicted while pregnant.

SIGNS AND SYMPTOMS

If you see a person with a definite yellow-orange hue, lock up your carrots if you want to keep them for yourself. Eating several pounds of carrots a day will turn your hands and the soles of your feet orange, and give the rest of your skin a yellowy tint. This is because the carotene in carrots gets deposited in the outermost layer of the skin (carotene is the chemical that makes carrots orange). This symptom of carrot addiction is actually harmless.

The more troubling symptom for addicts is the simple but unstoppable desire to consume carrots. Published case studies detail the plight of patients who resorted to stealing to satisfy their cravings. Other sufferers constantly think about carrots, and plot their days around when and where to get their next "fix."

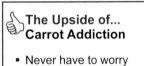

**The Upside of...
Carrot Addiction**

- Never have to worry about getting enough vitamins.
- Much safer than heroin addiction.
- Possible x-ray vision from eating so many carrots.

DIAGNOSIS AND TREATMENT

There's no formal diagnosis as of yet for carrot addiction. But suffice it to say, if you regularly eat ten pounds of carrots a day, no one will deny that you are a carrot addict.

As for treatment, therapy has been found effective in lessening the psychological craving for carrots.

PROGNOSIS

With proper treatment it is possible to conquer carrot addiction. But even if you can't kick the habit, eating copious amounts of carrots will not kill you.

PREVALENCE

No one is exactly sure how many carrot addicts are out there. Undoubtedly, many addicts are embarrassed by their habit and do not come forward for help.

HOW TO AVOID IT

Eat celery!

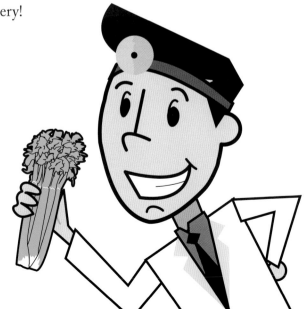

NOTABLE CASES

- One of the patients featured in Ludek and Karel Cerny's study was a man who took up eating carrots after he quit smoking. The man's wife suggested he munch on the carrots as a distraction from his nicotine craving. It worked, but soon the man was consuming up to five bunches of carrots a day. He did end up getting control of the addiction, but only when a carrot shortage in eastern Europe cut off his supply.

- Another one of the Cernys' patients—a thirty-eight-year-old woman from Prague—would not have been stopped by any carrot shortage. This patient took to stealing bags of carrots from the horse paddocks at a local racetrack. As if stealing snacks from thoroughbreds wasn't desperate enough, this patient also saved her carrot peels for use in "emergency" situations.

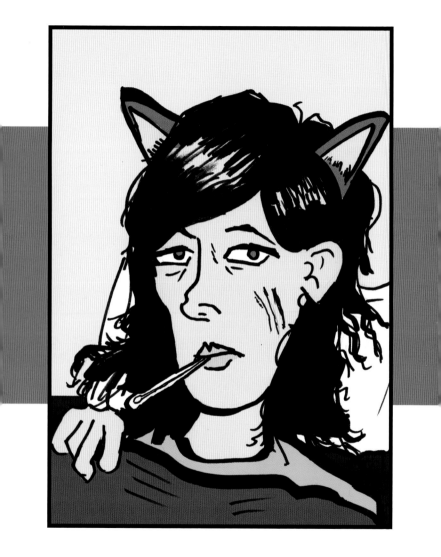

CAT SCRATCH FEVER

And you thought cat scratch fever was just the name of a bad Ted Nugent song, eh? Well, turns out it's totally real. One minute you're playing with a cute and cuddly kitten and the next the little fucker bites or scratches you. Happens all the time, right? But if that pussycat is infected with the bacteria that cause cat scratch fever, then look out.

WHAT IS IT?

Cat scratch fever is caused by the bacteria *Bartonella henselae*. It's transmitted through scratches and bites from an infected cat—although it also can be caught through touching the whites of an infected cat's eyes and then rubbing your own eyes (although, who the hell goes around touching the whites of a cat's eyes?!). You also may contract it by petting an infected cat's fur and rubbing your eyes, because while the bacteria live in a cat's saliva, cats lick their fur, paws, and claws frequently, leaving traces of the bacteria on those parts of their bodies. So you don't need to be swapping spit with a cat to get infected.

ORIGINS

Cat scratch disease was first described by the French physician and pediatrician Robert Debre in 1931. But it wasn't until 1992 that the bacteria *Bartonella henselae* were isolated as the cause of the infection.

WHAT CAUSES IT?

Researchers think cats may initially acquire the *Bartonella henselae* virus from fleas, but to date that hasn't been proven. What is known is that the bacteria are passed from cat to human when an infected cat bites or scratches your skin, and less often after touching an infected cat's fur or the whites of its eyes.

> ### ✍ The Upside of...
> ### Cat Scratch Fever
>
> - The real reason cats are not man's best friend.
> - Proof that it's never a good idea to let a cat lick your open wounds.
> - The only disease to have spawned a Billboard Top 100 single.

SIGNS AND SYMPTOMS

You may have cat scratch disease if you have:

- ☒ A bump or blister at the site of a cat scratch or bite. Such sores may take three to ten days to appear after being scratched or bitten.
- ☒ A cat scratch or bite that doesn't heal in the normal amount of time
- ☒ Redness around a scratch or bite that continues to worsen
- ☒ Fever that lasts for several days
- ☒ Swelling of lymph nodes near the injury
- ☒ General fatigue, headache, and achiness that go on for several days

DIAGNOSIS AND TREATMENT

A blood test can confirm whether you have *Bartonella henselae* antibodies, a sure sign you have cat scratch disease.

In most cases, cat scratch fever clears up in a matter of weeks without any special treatment. In some instances, antibiotics are prescribed—such as when patients have painful infected lymph nodes for a period of two to three months after the infection.

Cat scratch fever is more serious in people who have suppressed immune systems—such as AIDS patients. For these patients, antibiotics are just about always necessary to fight the infection.

By the way, there is no way to treat your cat for carrying *Bartonella henselae*. The bacteria are not harmful to cats and only become a problem when they infect humans.

PROGNOSIS

Most people infected with cat scratch fever make a complete recovery. It's only a serious concern in patients with suppressed immune systems.

PREVALENCE

Since cases of cat scratch fever often don't require medical attention, it is difficult to say exactly how many people contract it each year. But some estimates put the annual infection rate in the U.S. at 24,000 people.

HOW TO AVOID IT

Get a dog!

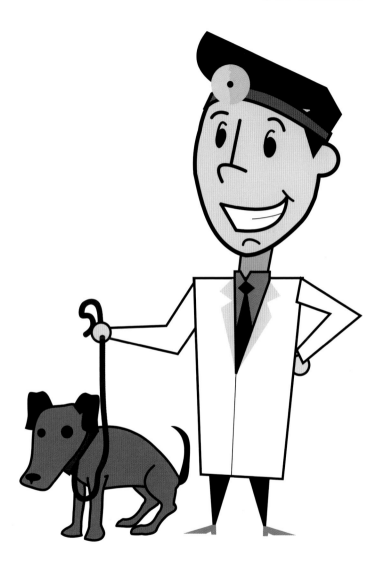

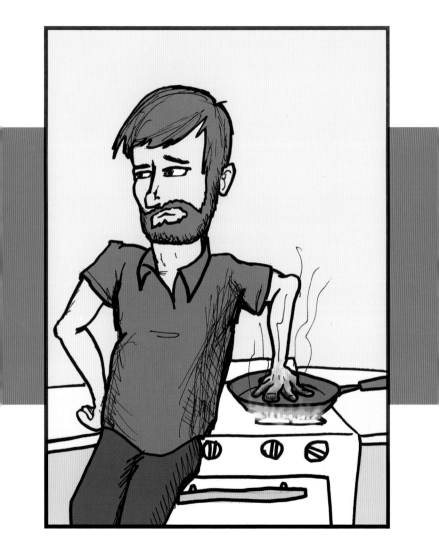

CONGENITAL INSENSITIVITY TO PAIN WITH ANHIDROSIS (CIPA)

Pain may be annoying, but we feel it for a reason. That reason, of course, is that there's something wrong, and the body wants you to know it. Smash your finger with a hammer and it hurts—a lot. That's your body telling you that you have shitty aim. Okay, just kidding. The throbbing pain you feel is for your own protection; it's the nervous system's way of making sure you take note of your injury and do something about it.

Equally annoying is the fact that we humans are only comfortable in a fairly small range of temperatures. When the mercury soars too high, we complain of the heat and desperately fan ourselves while we sweat through our clothes. Conversely, when the temperature drops below our comfort level, we bitch and moan through chattering teeth about how cold we are.

But what if you didn't feel any pain? And what if you weren't sensitive to heat or cold? Sounds pretty good, eh? Well, it isn't. Just ask someone with congenital insensitivity to pain with anhidrosis (or CIPA for short).

WHAT IS IT?

People with CIPA have damaged nervous systems, which result in their sensory perceptions running amok. While they are able to feel pressure on the skin (such as tickling or hugs), they cannot feel pain. In addition, CIPA patients are unable to sweat, and thus their bodies cannot regulate their internal temperature (*anhidrosis* means "absence of sweat").

CIPA is actually part of a family of genetic nervous system disorders called hereditary sensory and autonomic neuropathies (HSAN), and is sometimes referred to as HSAN IV.

> **The Upside of... CIPA**
>
> - After reading this chapter, you'll never be happier to feel pain and sweat like a pig.
> - Makes getting a root canal feel like a treat.
> - No child should have to suffer like this. No joke.

ORIGINS

CIPA was first described in medical literature in 1932 and was officially listed as a disorder in 1983.

WHAT CAUSES IT?

Patients with CIPA are born with the disorder. It is caused by a mutation of the NTRK1 gene, which is crucial to the development of nerves related to feeling pain, heat, and cold. CIPA is an autosomal recessive disorder, which means that a child must receive one copy of the mutated gene from each parent.

SIGNS AND SYMPTOMS

Children with CIPA typically exhibit the following symptoms:

- ☒ Inability to feel pain.
- ☒ Bumps, bruises, cuts, and scrapes do not bother a small child. Even broken bones and serious burns may go unnoticed.
- ☒ Joint problems due to overwork.
- ☒ In infants, teething becomes a nightmare, as children are likely to gnaw on their fingers until they bleed or actually chew through their tongues.
- ☒ Eye injuries are very common in children with CIPA. Many wear protective goggles to prevent them from accidentally scratching and damaging their corneas.
- ☒ The inability to sweat puts CIPA patients at grave risk of heat stroke, which can cause brain damage or even result in death. Inability to feel cold increases the risk of hypothermia.
- ☒ A high percentage of CIPA patients who live past age three suffer from mental retardation.

DIAGNOSIS AND TREATMENT

CIPA is so rare that getting a diagnosis can be difficult. However, a child experiencing the signs and symptoms above is likely to have the disorder.

There is no cure for CIPA—all patients can do for now is manage it as best they can. And because CIPA is present at birth, many of the management techniques are aimed at preventing children from accidentally maiming themselves.

- ☒ Because they can't sweat, patients must be kept in an environment that's not too hot and not too cold—usually between 65 to 72 degrees Fahrenheit. Patients must avoid direct sunlight. In most cases, swimming is the only exercise that's safe for a CIPA patient to perform.
- ☒ Kids with CIPA are taught that when they see blood, they must stop what they're doing and seek help. "Child proofing" takes on a new meaning when a kid with CIPA is in the house. Absolutely anything sharp or hot must be stashed away or securely covered to prevent injury to the child.
- ☒ Goggles or protective eyewear are often used to prevent children from scratching their eyes and severely damaging their corneas.
- ☒ In infants with CIPA, teething is a huge problem. Children regularly chew their lips until they bleed and some have even been known to chew through their tongues. In many CIPA cases, most of the teeth are removed and the child has to be fed through a feeding tube.

PROGNOSIS

Overheating kills more than half of all children with CIPA before age three. Those who do live beyond three often don't make it to adulthood. Infections from untreated wounds can lead to complications and death. For example, cases have been documented in which a child's appendix has burst without the child showing any sign of a problem. A high percentage of people with CIPA who live beyond three suffer from mental retardation, often because of frequent fevers that hamper proper brain development.

PREVALENCE

There are roughly a few dozen cases of CIPA in the United States. Japan has the highest number of cases due to the fact that genetic disorders are more common in homogeneous societies.

HOW TO AVOID IT

As with any genetic disorder, it's impossible to avoid getting CIPA. Anyone with the condition was, unfortunately, born with it.

NOTABLE CASES

CIPA has been featured in storylines on both the *Grey's Anatomy* and *House* TV shows.

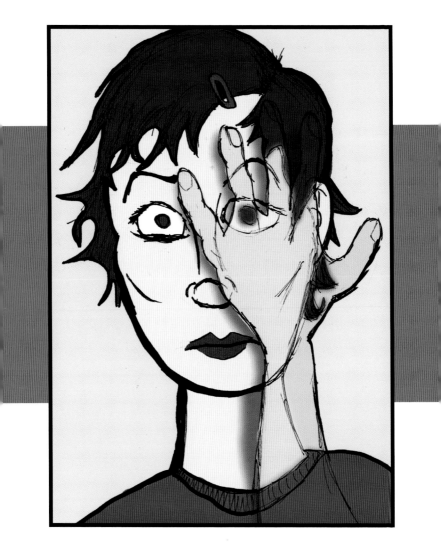

COTARD'S SYNDROME

"If you're dead, how am I speaking with you right now?" You have to admit that the question the doctor standing in front of you has just asked is a fair one. "I don't know," you say, "But I know that I'm dead." The doctor asks you to put your hand on your chest and feel your beating heart. You do as he asks, and indeed you feel the telltale thump-thump of your ticker ticking away. "That proves nothing," you say to the doctor. "All I know is that I'm dead."

Welcome to the wild world of Cotard's syndrome (aka, Cotard's delusion or walking corpse syndrome).

WHAT IS IT?

Cotard's syndrome is a neuropsychiatric disorder in which patients display a range of delusions: thinking that they are dead, that they do not exist, that their organs or blood is missing, that they have no soul, that they are decomposing, or that they are immortal. Patients persist in believing these delusions despite concrete evidence to the contrary (e.g., recognizing they have a beating heart, yet still insisting they are dead).

ORIGINS

Cotard's syndrome is named after the French neurologist, psychiatrist, and military surgeon Jules Cotard. In 1880 Cotard delivered a paper describing a forty-three-year-old female patient who displayed a bewildering array of symptoms. The woman believed she had no brain or nerves, that neither God nor the devil existed, that she did not need food or water, and that she would live forever. In 1882, Cotard named the condition *le délire de negation*, or "negation delirium."

The Upside of...
Cotard's Syndrome

- Finally, an excuse not to pay taxes.
- Get to go to your own funeral.
- Skip cleaning the house, making the bed, being faithful to your lover . . . screw it; you're dead, after all.

WHAT CAUSES IT?

Severe depression is the most common cause of Cotard's, but it's also been linked to strokes, dementia, and brain injuries, as well as to schizophrenia and bipolar disorder. Some researchers also believe that lesions on certain parts of the brain can also cause Cotard's. It tends to strike most in older people.

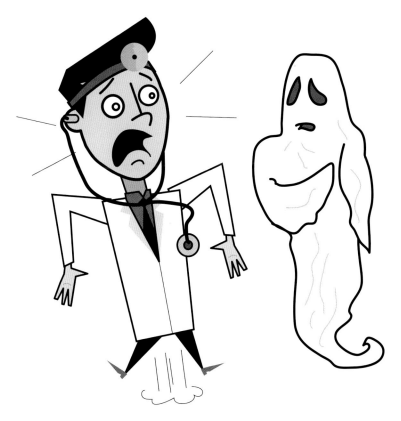

Many researchers believe Cotard's is related to Capgras syndrome, another delusional disorder. Patients with Capgras believe their friends and relatives have been replaced with impostors. It is thought that the syndromes stem from a neurological disconnect between the areas of the brain that associate faces with emotions. It is possible that in Cotard's people don't recognize their own face, thus leading them to believe they are dead. Still, there is debate about how much the delusions stem from physical factors and how much can be attributed to psychological causes.

SIGNS AND SYMPTOMS

As noted above, a person with Cotard's is likely to believe that he or she is dead or dying, putrefying, has no soul, or is missing organs or his or her blood. The patient persists in these delusions despite being shown evidence to the contrary. Cotard's sufferers may even recognize that their belief is illogical, yet they cannot be shaken out of their delusion.

DIAGNOSIS AND TREATMENT

The first step in diagnosing Cotard's syndrome is to rule out any other factors that could lead a patient to display such odd symptoms (like he or she is just batshit crazy!). Since depression is such a large factor in most Cotard's cases, treating a patient's depression is usually the most common course of action. However, drugs have been shown to do little to help stop the delusions. Patients have responded much better to electroconvulsive shock therapy. Several cases have been reported in which after shock therapy the patient's delusions entirely stopped. Electroshock therapy was usually followed by a course of antipsychotic drugs, such as olanzapine.

PROGNOSIS

Cotard's is difficult to treat, and the patient may struggle with it his or her entire life.

PREVALENCE

Researchers don't have a good idea of the prevalence of Cotard's.

HOW TO AVOID IT

Aside from avoiding brain injuries, there's not much you can actively do to prevent developing Cotard's.

NOTABLE CASES

- In 2004, psychiatrists from the School of Medicine at Turkey's Trakya University reported the case of a twenty-seven-year-old man who was referred to them for evaluation. The man, called Mr. G in the study, complained of headaches, shortness of breath, and, most shockingly, claimed that his stomach was missing. He had stopped eating solid food, dropping from a weight of 165 pounds to 139 pounds in a month's time. Mr. G's parents noted to doctors that their son's mood had deteriorated over the previous couple of years, and that he'd become withdrawn socially and was failing at his job. Both cardiologic and gastrointestinal examinations showed no physical cause of his symptoms. Doctors diagnosed Mr. G with schizophreniform disorder, a short-term form of schizophrenia. He was given antipsychotic drugs and was admitted to the psychiatric clinic.

Within a few hours of being admitted, he'd escaped from the hospital and was picked up by police some time later three to four miles away. His reason for escaping, he said, was because there was no oxygen in the clinic. The following morning, Mr. G attempted to escape through the ventilation system in the clinic bathroom. He was given a higher dosage of antipsychotics. But after two weeks of medication Mr. G had shown no improvement. A course of electroconvulsive therapy (more commonly known as shock treatment) was tried. After a week of the electro treatments, Mr. G made marked improvements. After a total of twelve treatments, his Cotard's symptoms had remitted. Soon after, he was released from the hospital and was able to return to normal social functions.

- Also in 2004, a twenty-four-year-old nurse—named LU in the study—was admitted to the National Hospital for Neurology and Neurosurgery in London due to seizures. She was diagnosed with epilepsy and spent a month in the hospital. A neuropsychological profile performed during her hospital stay showed problems beyond epilepsy. During an examination she repeatedly told a doctor she was dead and that she had died two weeks earlier—the same time she was admitted to the hospital. She asked if the hospital was heaven. She also told doctors she was unable to kiss her boyfriend because "it feels strange—although I know that he loves me." She complained of dizziness, hallucinated she was hearing disco music, said she felt running water on her left forearm, and claimed that the walls were moving. Over the next few days she became less certain she was dead, and within a week, the delusion had gone away entirely.

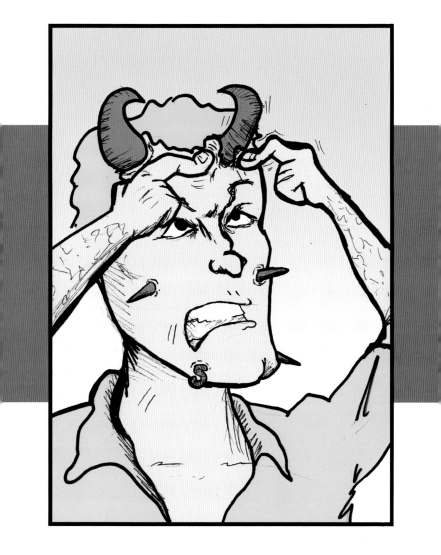

CUTANEOUS HORN

"What is *that*?!" Your friend is staring intently at your ear, making a face like he's just drunk some spoiled milk. "What is what?" you reply. "That! That weird, freaky thing growing out of the top of your ear?" You lift your hand up to your head and caress the top of your right ear. You feel a bump. "Oh, that," you say. "It just appeared there. I guess I should get it checked out." Days go by and you're busy, so you don't call the dermatologist. But every morning when you wake, it's clear that the "bump" on your ear is bigger. When you get your morning coffee, people stare. Children move away from you after glancing at your head. Are you turning into the devil? Why is a horn growing out of your head?

Never fear: dark forces are not at work and you're not turning into Beelzebub. You have cutaneous horn.

WHAT IS IT?

Cutaneous horn (also known by the Latin name *cornu cutaneum*, which means "horn of skin") is a rare skin condition in which horn-like growths protrude from the skin. Although it looks like bone, the horn is actually a dense tumorous collection of keratin, the protein in skin that gives it its strength and flexibility (keratin also is the protein of which fingernails are made).

ORIGINS

No one researcher is credited with "discovering" cutaneous horn. The condition has almost certainly been around for thousands of years, and is more than likely responsible for several myths of horn-like creatures throughout history.

One of the earliest known cases is that of a Welsh woman named Margaret Gryffith, who in the late sixteenth century was popular on the London stage thanks to her four-inch horn. Roughly 200 years later, in 1791, the London surgeon Everard Home wrote of the condition. Since then, it has baffled doctors and medical researchers.

WHAT CAUSES IT?

Cutaneous horns form on the surface of the skin due to an overgrowth of the skin protein keratin. The keratin that makes up the horn is actually dead, and the horn itself is a symptom of what's really going on below the skin. The horns stem from a variety of usually benign lesions. They also may grow out of warts, scars, and cysts. However, in about one-third of cases, the horns grow from premalignant or malignant lesions.

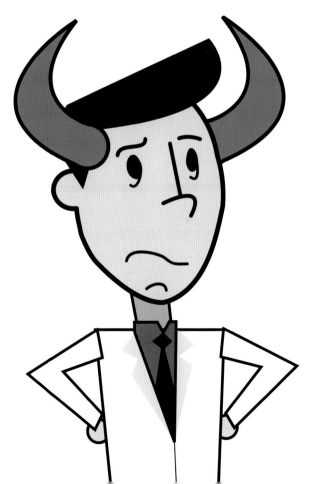

Typically, the horns grow on areas of the skin regularly exposed to the sun, such as the face, ears, nose, arms, and hands, but also have been documented on other body parts (including the penis!).

Researchers don't know what causes the horns to grow, but many believe that exposure to radiation from the sun is one of the primary triggers.

SIGNS AND SYMPTOMS

Let's face it—you'll probably know if you have cutaneous horn without having to read a list of symptoms. But just in case there's any question whether the growth on your head is a cutaneous horn—and that you're not turning into a unicorn—here are the symptoms:

- ☒ The horn-like growth may be rough and scaly, or it may be smooth and polished.
- ☒ Horns may be anywhere from a few millimeters in length to several centimeters. In a few cases, horns have grown to very large sizes—in excess of 50 cm.
- ☒ Usually cone-shaped, horns have also been documented in twisted shapes and protruding from the skin at an angle.
- ☒ The horn is usually yellowish in color, but also may be brown or almost black.

DIAGNOSIS AND TREATMENT

The horn should be surgically removed. In some cases, the horn will grow back after it is excised. If the growth was from a benign lesion, no further treatment is necessary. When the horn has grown from a malignant lesion, the lesion also has to be treated.

PROGNOSIS

The horns may be disgusting, but, in most cases, a complete recovery is possible.

PREVALENCE

Lighter skinned people are more inclined to get cutaneous horns, although they have been documented in darker-skinned people as well. It strikes older people more often, with the majority of cases seen in people in their sixties and seventies. It shows no predilection for gender, affecting both men and women at equal rates.

The Upside of...
Cutaneous Horn

- Get to yell out, "Who's horny? I am!"
- Moonlight as the devil at a haunted house at Halloween time.
- When people look at you funny, say, "My dad was a rhino."

HOW TO AVOID IT

Keep your fingers (and toes) crossed…. There's no way to avoid getting cutaneous horn. You just have to hope your body doesn't flip out.

However, as sun exposure seems to encourage horn growth, the usual sun precautions should be followed to diminish your chances of getting cutaneous horn (i.e., slather on the sunscreen and keep your face and body screened from direct sun).

NOTABLE CASES

- Dede Koswara—the Tree Man

Far and away the most famous case of cutaneous horn is that of Dede Koswara, the "Tree Man" of Indonesia. After he cut himself as a teenager, a small wart formed on the injury. Over time, the wart spread and grew. Eventually, Koswara's hands and feet were engulfed by horns that grew so long that he appeared to have gnarled tree roots growing at the end of his limbs. The growths partially covered his face and neck as well. His wife left him, he lost his job, and he took to performing as a circus freak to help support his children. But in 2007, at age thirty-five, the root problem (heh heh) of Koswara's condition was diagnosed by an American dermatologist. He suffers from a rare immune deficiency in which the body is unable to check the growth of warts caused by the human papilloma virus (HPV). In 2008, Koswara underwent surgery to remove four pounds of horny growths. Today, Koswara is thirty-seven and has nearly full use of his hands and feet for the first time in more than twenty years.

- **The Horny Granny**

In 2007, Weird News sections of newspapers the world over ran the story of a ninety-five-year-old Chinese woman from Zhanjiang City, in Southeastern China, who had a five-inch horn growing from her forehead. According to reports, the horn began to grow in 2003, and the woman had first thought it was a mole. She sought treatment for the horn because it was starting to obstruct her vision.

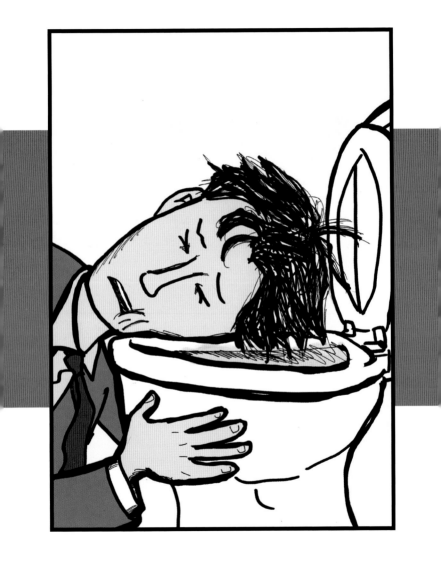

CYCLIC VOMITING SYNDROME (CVS)

Here we go again . . . The last few times you felt this nauseous, you vomited for four days straight! No one should be so familiar with the intricate pattern of cracks in the tiles around their toilet—but when you throw up eight times an hour for several days, you spend a lot of time curled up on the bathroom floor!

The first time this happened, you were sure you just had food poisoning. But when several hours stretched into several days, you knew some bad shellfish wasn't the problem. Your doctor said it was a stomach flu, and lo and behold, you recovered and returned to your normal routine. But then it happened again, and again, and again. . . . And now here you are, yet one more time, back in the bathroom unable to stop hurling.

Unfortunately for you, it appears that your problem is more than just a weak stomach. You very well may have cyclic vomiting syndrome.

WHAT IS IT?

Cyclic vomiting syndrome (CVS) is a disorder in which patients experience drawn-out episodes of extreme nausea and vomiting with no obvious cause. Between episodes, the patient leads a healthy normal life.

ORIGINS

CVS was first described in medical literature in 1882 by the English pediatrician Dr. Samuel Gee.

WHAT CAUSES IT?

No one knows what causes CVS. However, CVS researchers have compiled a variety of triggers that may prompt an episode, including:

- ☒ Colds, flu, and other infections
- ☒ Emotional stress or anxiety
- ☒ Eating certain foods
     (chocolate and cheese are often cited)
- ☒ Overeating

The Upside of...
Cyclic Vomiting Syndrome

- Make a convincing remake of *The Exorcist*.
- Lose weight; no gym membership required.
- Look on the bright side: your next hangover will feel like nothing compared to this.

☒ Eating close to bedtime
☒ Motion sickness
☒ Hot weather
☒ Menstruation

SIGNS AND SYMPTOMS

CVS occurs in four phases: symptom-free interval phase, prodrome phase, vomiting phase, and recovery phase.

Symptom-Free Interval Phase

The period between flare-ups of CVS.

Prodrome Phase

In this phase, nausea—and sometimes stomach pain—signals that a bout of vomiting is on its way. It can last anywhere from a few minutes up to several hours. Sometimes, a round of vomiting may be held off by taking medicine during the prodrome phase.

Vomiting Phase

This phase consists of ongoing nausea and prolonged episodes of vomiting, lasting usually from several hours to a few days, but can go on for up to three weeks.

Recovery Phase

The nausea and vomiting stop, appetite returns, and the person is able to resume his or her normal life.

Along with the above phases, the following symptoms are commonly seen in patients during bouts of CVS:

- ☒ Abdominal pain
- ☒ Dizziness
- ☒ Sensitivity to light
- ☒ Headache
- ☒ Dehydration
- ☒ Listlessness
- ☒ Pallor
- ☒ Tooth decay from the acid in vomit
- ☒ Peptic esophagitis (inflammation of the esophagus)
- ☒ Hematemesis (the esophagus becomes so irritated it bleeds, and the blood is mixed with the vomit)
- ☒ Mallory-Weiss tear (a tear in the esophagus where it connects to the stomach)

DIAGNOSIS AND TREATMENT

Diagnosis of CVS is complicated by the fact that there is no definitive test for it. Tests may be performed to rule out other problems, but a diagnosis of CVS is based on the patient's history.

Treatment depends on the severity of the CVS episode. At the very least, most patients require a quiet, dark space in which to recover from bouts of nausea and vomiting. Anti-nausea and anti-vomiting medications may help relieve symptoms. In the recovery phase, it is necessary to replace lost fluids and electrolytes to reinvigorate the body.

Hospitalization may be required if the patient becomes dehydrated. At the hospital, fluids and medication may be given intravenously.

Long term hope for treatment may lie in the connection between CVS and migraine. Researchers have noticed links between the two afflictions, and children who outgrow CVS in their teens are much more likely to experience migraines as adults. In addition, children with CVS often have a family history of migraines.

PROGNOSIS

There is no treatment for CVS.

PREVALENCE

CVS may affect as many as one in fifty children, according to the renowned Mayo Clinic. It is believed to affect both sexes equally. It used to be thought of mainly as a pediatric disease, but can occur at any age.

HOW TO AVOID IT

There's no way to avoid getting CVS.

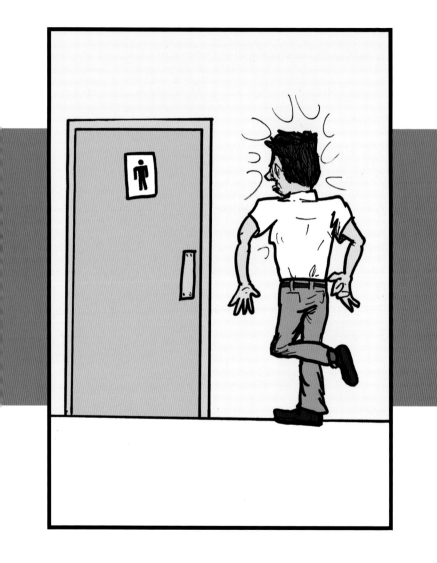

DEVELOPMENTAL TOPOGRAPHICAL DISORIENTATION

It's happening again. You've left the house with the simple intention of going to the park for a walk. You went out the front door, turned left, walked one block, crossed the street and now . . . and now . . . and now you're utterly dumbfounded about which way to go. *The park should be right there! Shouldn't it?*

You'd be in a panic right now, except that this happens all the time. Driving anywhere is a total disaster. If you didn't have a GPS unit in the car, you wouldn't make it to and from the supermarket!

You may think you just have a bad sense of direction, but that's not the real problem. What you have is a developmental brain disorder called topographical disorientation.

WHAT IS IT?

People with topographical disorientation cannot form mental maps of their surroundings. They're able to recognize landmarks, but they're unable to orient themselves in relation to these points. For example, a person may recognize he's standing outside his house, but have no idea how to navigate from that spot to the church five blocks away that he's attended since childhood. Because those with the condition never developed the ability to make these mental maps, they've usually spent their whole lives coping with getting lost very easily.

ORIGINS

Developmental topographical disorientation was first described in 2008 by a group of Canadian neuroscientists and neuropsychologists. In an article in the medical journal *Neuropsychologia*, the authors described the "first case of a patient with topographical disorientation in the absence of any structural lesion and with intact sensory and intellectual function." The article documented the case of Patient 1, a forty-three-year-old woman from Vancouver who needed help from her family and friends to navigate even around the neighborhood where she'd lived her entire life. After a battery of tests, the researchers concluded that Patient 1's navigational problems were due to the fact that she couldn't form cognitive maps. Since the publication of the article, its lead researcher, Giuseppe Iaria of the

University of Calgary, has found hundreds of other people with problems similar to Patient 1.

WHAT CAUSES IT?

Brain injuries or improper brain development can certainly lead to impaired navigational ability. In addition, brain lesions or stroke may affect the brain's capacity to recall and process information that helps us navigate our surroundings. Attention and memory disorders also may hamper our ability to find our way.

However, topographical disorientation also appears in people who show no signs of brain injury or cognitive impairment. In cases where a patient is otherwise healthy, researchers believe the cause of topographical disorientation is the patient's inability to form so-called "cognitive maps" of his or her environment. To understand the causes better, it helps to know how the brain functions when we navigate.

The Upside of...
Developmental Topographical Disorientation

- Always have an excuse for being late.
- Get out of being the navigator on long car trips.
- Have a convenient excuse to ask good-looking strangers for help getting where you're going.

As it turns out, finding your way around is a complex cognitive exercise. To navigate between two points, your brain relies on memory, perception, and decision-making; actually, it relies on two different kinds of memory: procedural memory and spatial memory. These two forms of memory hold the key to topographical disorientation.

Procedural memory is what we use when we follow routes with which we're very familiar—ones that require almost no attention from us to get where we're going. When navigating an environment with which we're not as familiar, we use spatial memory, a complex process of making connections between landmarks and our place in relation to those landmarks. So if you visit a new town, for example, you will know where your hotel is. When you walk to a restaurant, you take note of other landmarks you pass and mentally plot their relation to the hotel. As you move around the town more, you start to relate all of the landmarks you encounter to each other, making a cognitive map of this new environment. As you can see, being able to create a cognitive map is a more reliable way to navigate than using procedural memory, which is only useful once you're very familiar with your surroundings. Researchers believe that people with topographical disorientation are unable to make these cognitive maps.

Why people cannot form these cognitive maps remains a mystery. One area of the brain that researchers think plays a role in the formation of cognitive maps is the hippocampus, which is known to be an important center of memory and navigation.

SIGNS AND SYMPTOMS

When a patient is unable to find his or her way out of a paper bag, he or she has topographical disorientation! But seriously, a person with developmental topographical disorientation gets lost performing even the simplest navigational exercises.

DIAGNOSIS AND TREATMENT

A diagnosis of developmental topographical disorientation is made after other factors that may cause one to get lost are ruled out. If you have no other neurological issues or brain injuries, you get lost pretty much all the time no matter where you are, and you've had the problem for a long time, you probably have developmental topographical disorientation.

As for treatment, in the case of Patient 1, after six weeks of working with Iaria for an hour a week, she was able to reduce the time it took her to make a cognitive map of a virtual reality world from thirty-two minutes to five minutes. Iaria believes this shows that people with topographical disorientation can at least become *better* at making cognitive maps, even if they'll never be ace navigators.

THE HYPOCHONDRIAC'S HANDBOOK

What it takes is practice. Why they never developed the ability to make these maps in the first place remains a mystery.

PROGNOSIS

With treatment, people's ability to navigate can improve, but there is no cure for the condition. People with developmental topographical disorientation will always have to be conscious of not getting lost.

PREVALENCE

No one knows how many people have developmental topographical disorientation. Iaria and his colleagues have set up a Web site—www.gettinglost.ca—where you can take an online test to assess your navigational skills. Iaria hopes this will help him identify how prevalent the condition is.

HOW TO AVOID IT

If you or your child displays signs of developmental disorientation, see a neurologist immediately. You also should contact Giuseppe Iaria at his Web site: www.gettinglost.ca.

NOTABLE CASES

- Sharon Roseman

Sharon Roseman isn't famous. But the sixty-two-year-old, who lives outside Denver, has helped put a public face on topographical disorientation. Roseman's condition began when she was five, after playing a game in which she was blindfolded and spun in a circle. Since that day, she's hopelessly confused whenever she encounters a bend in a street or even a curve in a hallway. Roseman's condition has the interesting symptom that upon encountering such changes in direction, everything in her vision shifts 90 degrees. For example, if she's driving in her car, a store that should be on her right appears in front of her. Roseman is actually able to stop the symptoms by closing her eyes and spinning in place—yet she admits such a course of action is not always feasible in public.

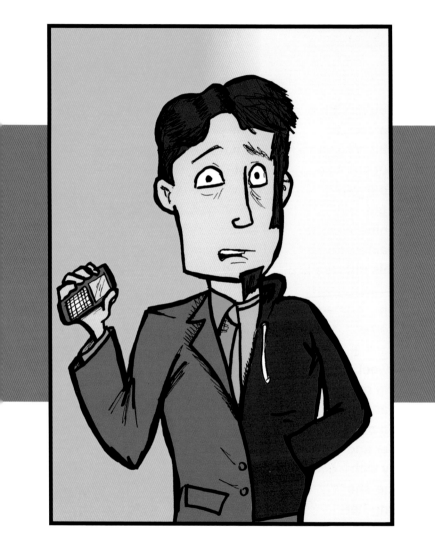

DISSOCIATIVE FUGUE

You're sitting in your living room listening to the person seated across from you say some really weird shit. You swear you've never met this person before, but she's telling you that she's *your wife*. What the…? Your wife!? You *have* a wife, and she's in the kitchen right now, getting you and your mysterious guest some iced tea. The woman across from you looks pained. You feel bad for her, but you wonder how long this nutcase is planning to stay.

The woman reaches into her handbag and pulls out some photos. "So you don't remember your children—Jack and Vanessa?" She hands you a photo of some sweet smiling kids, who you must admit bear a passing resemblance to you. "Look at this one," she says, handing you another snapshot. "This is you and me on our deck—six years ago." You take the photo from her and gaze at it. The man in the photo sitting cheerily with a beer in his hand has your face; the woman in the shot sitting on his knee is clearly the woman sitting here across from you now. Photoshop trickery? It doesn't look like it. But it sure as hell doesn't make any sense either.

The woman passes you another photo, and says, "Us, hiking in the Rockies." Again, it looks just like you. You look at her uncomprehendingly. How could this be?

"Who are you?" you stammer at this stranger as your head spins. "I am Nancy," she says wearily. "I am your wife."

Over the next hours you learn you've lived two lives. Not at the same time, like when spouses have affairs—or are secretly gay—and can be said to be leading double lives. Not like that at all. In your case, it's like the life you were leading suddenly ended, yet you started an entirely new life in the same body.

Nancy tells you that one day, five years ago, you kissed her and your two small kids goodbye, left your suburban Cincinnati home for your job as a corporate lawyer, and then vanished. Today, you're sitting in Southern California, where you've worked your way up to be an assistant manager at an agricultural company.

How could this have happened?

_____

WHAT IS IT?

Dissociative fugue (also known as dissociative amnesia) is a psychiatric disorder that wipes clean a person's memory, causing a complete loss of identity. While the majority of episodes are relatively short-lived—lasting from several hours to a few days—some cases have been known to last years. The condition is reversible, and, upon "awakening" from a fugue, a person usually remembers all of the previous details of his or her life. However, upon recovery, events from during the fugue state are forgotten, leaving victims to piece together what's happened to them while they were "living another life." Those suffering from dissociative fugue often travel or wander far from home while in the fugue state. Indeed the word fugue comes from the Latin word *fuga*, which means "flight."

ORIGINS

One of the first documented cases of dissociative fugue was that of Ansel Bourne. In January 1887, Bourne, a sixty-one-year-old preacher who was known to have suffered from amnesia-like symptoms in the past, traveled from his home in Greene, Rhode Island to Norristown, Pennsylvania. Once there, he opened a stationery and confection shop and took the name A. J. Brown. One morning in mid-March, however, Bourne woke up and was utterly mystified by his surroundings. He had no memory of the previous two months and still believed it was January, and that he was in Rhode Island.

**The Upside of...
Dissociative Fugue**

- See the world—albeit without remembering anything.
- Best excuse ever to break up with a lover.
- See what it literally means to walk a mile—or 1,000—in someone else's shoes.

Upon his return home, Bourne agreed to be studied by Richard Hodgson of the Society for Psychical Research and the famed Harvard psychologist and philosopher William James. The researchers put Bourne under hypnosis and discovered that he was able to switch between his own memories and those of A. J. Brown's, but neither personality had any knowledge of the other. Upon awakening from hypnosis, Bourne again assumed his "normal" personality as Ansel Bourne.

Bourne's case continues to have echoes today. Most notably, it is believed by many that Robert Ludlum named his famous amnesiac secret agent, Jason Bourne (made famous onscreen by Matt Damon), after Ansel Bourne.

Dissociative fugue is related to dissociative identity disorder (or multiple personality disorder). But whereas patients with dissociative identity disorder have recurring multiple personalities, sufferers of dissociative fugue do not necessarily adopt character traits from previous fugue states.

WHAT CAUSES IT?

Dissociative fugue is not precipitated by any medical or physical condition. It is a psychological response to severe trauma. The trauma may be in the form of overwhelming stress—from a divorce or financial woes, for example—or it can result from a physical injury. People who've lived through war, natural disasters, accidents, or other traumatic events are more prone to suffer from such fugues. The psyche seems to be seeking a way out of the stress, and, in response, shuts down a person's memory. It's also possible that the fugues are an attempt by the mind to shut out suicidal or homicidal impulses.

SIGNS AND SYMPTOMS

The major symptom of dissociative fugue, of course, is a complete loss of identity. The sufferer will function completely normally, with no loss of physical or mental capability, but will have no idea who he or she is.

In the fugue state, sufferers tend to travel—sometimes going great distances—and adopt new identities, complete with new jobs, new friends, new likes and dislikes, and even new families.

It is possible, as with Ansel Bourne, that a person may "snap" out of his or her fugue. A person may also slowly emerge from it, recalling a few memories at a time and slowly piecing together his or her non-fugue identity.

DIAGNOSIS AND TREATMENT

There's no laboratory test to diagnose dissociative fugue, but the first step in diagnosing it is to rule out any physical problems that could be causing the fugue state.

Treatment usually consists of psychotherapy to address any underlying stress that may be causing the fugue, and to help the patient learn what might trigger fugue episodes.

PROGNOSIS

It's possible to make a full recovery from dissociative fugue. Sometimes memories return all at once, as if the person were awakening from a dream and back into full consciousness. Other times a person can be jarred from a fugue when confronted with evidence of his or her past. Once back in their normal state, however, patients cannot remember events that occurred during the fugue. The confusion caused by having lived hours, days, months, or years, of which one has no memory, can lead to anger and depression among those with dissociative fugue.

PREVALENCE

According to the Merck Manual, dissociative fugue affects about .2 percent of people in the United States.

HOW TO AVOID IT

Seeing as stress is the main precipitating factor in bringing on the fugue state, it's best to do all you can to manage the stress in your life. Certainly people who've lived through war or a natural disaster should seek help for any post-traumatic stress issues, as dissociative fugue is more common among those who've had these experiences. Additionally, with the help of a therapist, patients may be able to learn what situations and emotional states trigger their fugues.

NOTABLE CASES

- **Agatha Christie**

On the evening of December 3, 1926, the famed mystery writer Agatha Christie disappeared for eleven days. The thirty-six-year-old author was eventually discovered safe and sound at a hotel. She had checked in using the name Teresa Neele and had been living at the hotel since the day after she went missing. Although her picture was splashed across every newspaper in England, Christie apparently did not recognize her own face in print. When other hotel guests approached her, she laughed off the possibility she was the famed novelist. Nonetheless, the hotel contacted Christie's husband, who traveled to indentify her and bring her home. Christie eventually recovered, but her 1926 "disappearance" mystified her fans for years.

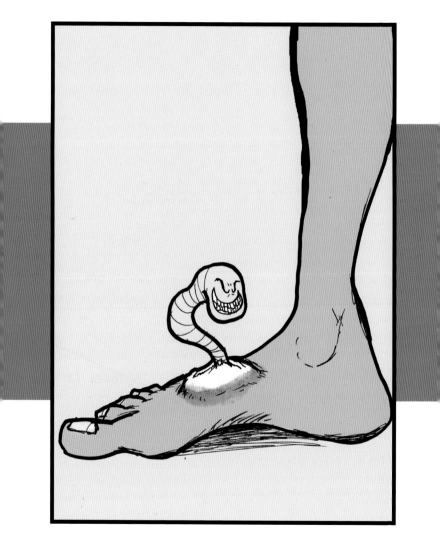

DRACUNCULIASIS
(GUINEA WORM DISEASE)

It's been about a year since you got back from your amazing trip to Africa. The safari in Kenya was great and South Africa was paradise. But West Africa was truly special, especially your time in Ghana. Ah, the beaches . . . The nightlife in Accra . . . You have your pictures and your memories for sure, but, as it turns out, you took home more than those from Ghana.

One morning you wake up and discover a blister on the top of your foot. *That's weird*, you think, *I don't recall any reason I'd have a blister there*. You hobble out of bed, and the pain in your foot is intense. Somehow you make it through the day at work, but, when you get home in the evening, the blister looks worse. You vow that if it's not better in the morning you'll call your doctor.

The next day you wake up and the blister is most definitely not better. Then the most disgusting thing you have ever seen in your life happens: the blister breaks open and a worm comes wriggling out of it. You scream, grab your head in horror, and run around the room in utter freak-out mode. You have dracunculiasis.

WHAT IS IT?

Dracunculiasis—more commonly known as Guinea worm disease (GWD)—is a parasitic infection caused by the parasite *Dracunculus medinensis*. GWD is contracted by drinking water infected with Guinea worm larvae. The female larvae grow in the body for about a year and then emerge as worms two to three feet in length.

ORIGINS

The name *dracunculiasis* is Latin for "affliction of little dragons," an apt, if inaccurate, description of the disease. It is actually one of the oldest documented human parasites. Researchers have found worms in 3,000-year-old Egyptian mummies. Accounts in Greek, Sanskrit, and Hebrew detail infection by the *Dracunculus medinensis*. The ancient Egyptian medical document from 1550 B.C. known as the Ebers Papyrus also details the effects of the disease and its treatment.

The first modern description of the disease was by the Bulgarian doctor Hristo Stambolski in 1877. While in exile in Yemen, Stambolski theorized that GWD was contracted by ingesting contaminated water.

WHAT CAUSES IT?

There is only one way to contract GWD, and that is by drinking contaminated water. You don't actually swallow a worm—the life cycle of the disease is way more disgusting than that!

Guinea worm larvae live in water where they are eaten by microscopic water fleas, called copepods. When you come along and drink the infested water, your stomach acid digests the tiny fleas, but not the larvae. The larvae travel through the digestive tract to the small intestine, where they proceed to burrow through the intestinal wall and into your body. Once in the body cavity, the male and female larvae mate, after which the male dies and is absorbed by the body. The female then burrows into tissue, usually next to long bones in the limbs. After a year of incubating inside its human host, the worm is anywhere from two to three feet long. It then attempts to leave the body by creating a blister on the surface of the skin and emerging through it. Soaking the affected limb or foot in water to soothe the burning of the blister causes the adult Guinea worm to release thousands of new larvae into the water, replicating the cycle of infection all over again.

SIGNS AND SYMPTOMS

- ☒ Pain and swelling in the area where the worm will emerge. In approximately 90 percent of cases, the worm comes out through a leg or a foot. The first symptoms also may be accompanied by fever.
- ☒ Within a few days or up to a couple of weeks later, a blister forms on the skin.

- ☒ Within 72 hours the blister becomes an open wound.
- ☒ The worm begins to emerge. It takes anywhere from ten days to a month for the worm to fully come out, during which time the pain can be intense.
- ☒ The worm can be coaxed out more quickly by wrapping it around a stick or grabbing it with gauze and pulling gently.

DIAGNOSIS AND TREATMENT

Combined with the above symptoms, a correct diagnosis of GWD is made when a worm pops through your skin.

There is no vaccine or treatment for Guinea worm disease. As mentioned above, the typical remedy is to wrap the worm around a stick and try to pull it out a little at a time—this can take anywhere from a few days to several weeks. One must be careful that the wound where the worm is leaving the body doesn't become infected.

PROGNOSIS

The blister that forms as the worm is readying to emerge is extremely painful. And removal of the worm causes intense discomfort. But once the worm is out, patients are able to return to their normal lives with no long-term problems.

PREVALENCE

The good news—for North Americans at least—is that GWD is currently found only in five African countries: Ghana, Mali, Niger, Nigeria, and Sudan. Just two cases have been reported in the U.S. since 1995, and both of those were in people who came to the States from Sudan.

An intense effort has been under way for many years now to eradicate GWD. Former president Jimmy Carter's foundation, the Carter Center, is at the forefront of the fight, and there is sincere hope that GWD will one day be the first parasitic disease ever eradicated from the face of the earth.

HOW TO AVOID IT

The easiest way to avoid getting GWD is to drink only filtered water. Water from underground sources—such as springs and wells—is also safe to drink.

The Upside of...
Dracunculiasis

- The ultimate souvenir of your African adventure—and it's free!
- Get the perfect pet; it never needs to be fed.
- Best excuse ever for not going to work: "I have to remove a two-foot-long worm that's growing inside my leg."

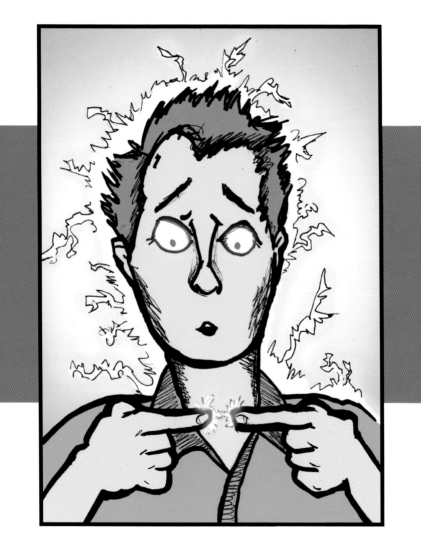

ELECTRIC HUMAN SYNDROME

We've all had the painfully annoying experience of shaking hands with a friend and getting zapped by a shock. Why does that happen? As you learned way back in high school physics, our bodies are nothing more than a collection of atoms—and atoms, in turn, are collections of positive and negative charges. So all it takes for us to get shocked is an imbalance between the positive and negative charges in our bodies. Such imbalances can arise from simple things, like walking across a rug or sitting in a plastic chair. What happens is electrons move from the chair or rug to your body, creating an overall electrical charge imbalance in your body. Now when you grab your friend's hand, electrons "jump" from you to him and you feel that movement of the electrons as a static shock. Okay, physics for dummies lesson over.

But what would happen if you didn't have to walk across a rug, or take off your sweater and touch a metal doorknob, or sit in a plastic chair to get a shock? For some people, none of these things are required to get a painful zap. They just seem to walk around getting shocked all the frigging time! These unfortunate folks are known as "electric people."

WHAT IS IT?

Electric humans spontaneously develop high voltage in their bodies due to an overall imbalance in their positive and negative electrical charges. As they make their way through their day, they are constantly getting zapped as their bodies try to balance out the charge.

ORIGINS

Reports of weird electrophysiological reactions in people have been around for centuries. But apparently scientists have thought they had better things to do than devote tons of time and money studying the phenomenon of electric humans. No formal research exists into this off-beat syndrome.

WHAT CAUSES IT?

Nobody knows. Most scientists deny the possibility that people can become electrified.

SIGNS AND SYMPTOMS

Constant shocks when touching other people or metal objects.

DIAGNOSIS AND TREATMENT

The first thing you should do if you suffer from electric human syndrome is eliminate the possibility that it's your clothes or shoes that's causing your problem. Once you've ruled out your wardrobe as the culprit, your options are somewhat limited. There's no cure for this problem, but you can take measures to reduce its negative effects. The best solution is probably to wear a thimble on your fingertip and constantly touch it to grounded metal objects, thus preventing you from getting shocked. Hey, it may look weird, but you also may start a new fashion trend among your friends!

> **The Upside of... Electric Human Syndrome**
>
> - Never worry about a blackout.
> - Convincingly use the pickup line, "You make me feel electric!"
> - Torture people you don't like by appearing friendly and constantly hugging—and shocking—them.

PROGNOSIS

There may be no cure for electric human syndrome, but it sure is cool!

PREVALENCE

There are no accurate statistics regarding the number of cases of electric human.

HOW TO AVOID IT

If you're prone to electric human syndrome, sorry, but you're stuck with it.

NOTABLE CASES

- In his 2002 book *Homemade Lightning*, R. A. Ford recounts two early documented occurrences of electric people. The first was reported in the 1838 edition of the journal *Annals of Electricity, Magnetism and Chemistry*. In this case a "lady of great respectability" became "suddenly and unconsciously charged with electricity" on the evening of January 25, 1837. She initially demonstrated her newfound powers by passing her hand over her brother's face, an act that sent sparks flying from her fingertips. She then repeated this amazing feat on several other willing participants. For the next three months, any conducting object she touched or came near to caused her to receive a shock. Picking up the scissors and needles in her sewing kit was a painful proposition, let alone cooking at her iron stove. The report stated that when the woman placed her finger within one-sixteenth of an inch from any metal object, "a spark that was heard, seen, and felt passed every second." Just as mysteriously as the condition arrived, it began to fade beginning at the end of February; by mid-May, it was completely gone.

- The second case was reported in a 1920 edition of *Science and Invention* magazine. This case involved thirty-four prisoners at the Clinton Prison in Dannemora, New York. The prisoners had become ill after eating canned salmon. Botulism was suspected, but the convicts all had some very strange side effects. The first sign of weirdness was when a prisoner in the infirmary crushed a piece of paper with his hands to throw in the trash, and, instead of being tossed, the paper stuck to his hand. Soon it was discovered that if an affected prisoner rubbed his hands together and placed one of them on a lightbulb, the filament inside would vibrate rapidly, move toward the hand, and then sparks would appear at the filament's bottom. Doctors investigating the strange case found that, as the patients recovered from the apparent botulism, their strange electrical powers declined and then disappeared. Despite the case of the electric prisoners attracting a lot of attention at the time, none of the investigators was ever able to understand the reason why they'd become electrified in the first place.

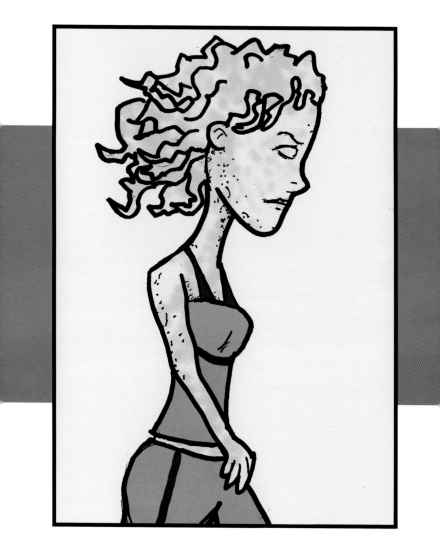

FIBRODYSPLASIA OSSIFICANS PROGRESSIVA
(FOP; STONE MAN SYNDROME)

Few disorders are as downright weird as fibrodysplasia ossificans progressiva (FOP). Imagine this: every time you fell down and bumped yourself (your arm, leg, or hand, for example) some of the muscles, tendons, and ligaments in the damaged area turned to bone. Or what if slowly over time you became a prisoner of your body, unable to move your limbs or your neck because the muscles and connective tissue that let those body parts move had ossified? It sounds like a curse from a fairy tale, but FOP is all too real.

WHAT IS IT?

The International Fibrodysplasia Ossificans Progressiva Association describes FOP as "One of the rarest, most disabling genetic conditions known to medicine." In FOP, muscles, tendons, ligaments, and other connective tissues are gradually replaced by bone. This extra-skeletal bone forms bridges across joints, restricting movement and effectively forming an extra skeleton—one that eventually makes the patient unable to move.

ORIGINS

The earliest documented cases of FOP are from the seventeenth and eighteenth centuries. French physician Guy Patin is credited with first describing FOP in 1692. In 1736, British surgeon John Freke was the first to declare that FOP was the result of a genetic error. Initially FOP was referred to as myositis ossificans progressiva, which means, "muscle turns progressively to bone." In the 1970s, the famed Johns Hopkins geneticist Victor A. McKusic renamed the disease fibrodysplasia ossificans progressiva to account for the fact that tissues other than muscle are affected by the condition.

WHAT CAUSES IT?

FOP is a genetic disease. In 2006, researchers at the University of Pennsylvania identified the gene responsible for FOP as ACVR1. The ACVR1 gene controls the growth and development of muscle and bone. A mutation of the ACVR1 gene is believed to be the cause of FOP. However, researchers don't yet know why the gene mutates.

Interestingly, the ACVR1 mutation in FOP patients is usually a new mutation of the gene. In other words, the majority of FOP patients come from families with no family history of FOP. Only a small number of cases are inherited from a parent with the ACVR1 mutation.

Most cases are diagnosed during childhood or in the teen years. Unfortunately, FOP is so rare that many cases are misdiagnosed as cancer or other, less serious, genetic diseases, such as aggressive juvenile fibromatosis.

SIGNS AND SYMPTOMS

In most FOP cases, the first symptom of the disorder is evident at birth: deformed big toes. The big toes of FOP

The Upside of...
FOP

- Not even the CIA could think of torture this bad.
- When a stiff neck is the least of your worries . . .
- The disease that's truly bad to the bone.

---

patients are unusually short and angled inwards toward the other toes. This first symptom is not usually a serious problem on its own, but it is a harbinger of much worse things to come.

More serious flare-ups of FOP typically occur before age ten. The excess bone growth starts in the neck and shoulders, continues into the arms and down the torso, and then into the legs and feet. As it progresses, FOP causes joints to become immobilized by interlocking ribbons of bone. Excess skeletal growth around the lungs may make it difficult for the patient to breathe. Ossified muscles around the mouth can make eating and drinking nearly impossible.

Bone growth may accelerate as a result of injuries to the muscles or connective tissues, such as from falling down or even from medical procedures. New bone grows at a rapid rate in the area of the trauma. Thus, surgically removing the misplaced bone only causes it to regrow even quicker.

DIAGNOSIS AND TREATMENT

FOP is frequently misdiagnosed as cancer, juvenile fibromatosis, or progressive osseous heteroplasia. The malformed big toe of an infant is usually a good indicator of FOP, and swellings on the head, back, and neck are also early indicators.

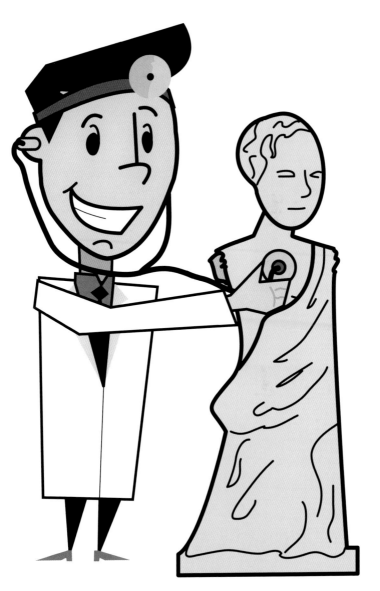

There is no known cure for FOP. However, one ongoing avenue of research into a cure involves the use of squalamine, an antibiotic derived from shark liver. In 2001, researchers began a clinical trial to test if squalamine was an effective way to slow bone growth in FOP cases.

While no cure exists, FOP symptoms can be somewhat managed by the use of steroids, anti-angiogenics (drugs that prevent the growth of blood vessels, which bones need to grow), anti-inflammatory drugs, and muscle relaxants.

PROGNOSIS

People with FOP are usually immobile by age 30. The average lifespan of FOP patients is 40 years.

PREVALENCE

FOP is believed to occur in one in every two million people worldwide. According to the International Fibrodysplasia Ossificans Progressiva Association, there are some 700 known cases around the globe, with 285 of those cases in the United States.

HOW TO AVOID IT

There's no way to prevent getting FOP.

NOTABLE CASES

- Harry Eastlack

By far the most famous case of FOP was that of Harry Eastlack, a Philadelphia man who lived with the condition for nearly forty years. Born in 1933, Eastlack's first symptoms of FOP occurred after he broke his leg at age five. His hip and knee stiffened after the accident, and bone began to replace the muscles of his thigh. In his twenties, Eastlack's vertebrae began to fuse. He died of pneumonia six days before his fortieth birthday. At the time of his death, the only part of his body that Eastlack could move was his lips. Before his death, however, he arranged for his body to be donated to science. Today, Eastlack's skeleton is on view at the famed Mütter Museum at the College of Physicians of Philadelphia.

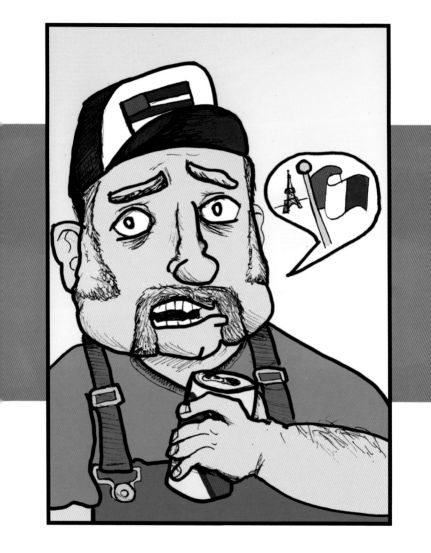

FOREIGN ACCENT SYNDROME

Where the hell am I?! you think, as you blink your eyes open and slowly focus them on the drab institutional walls of a hospital room. The last thing you remember, you were playing catcher in the company picnic softball game. Now you're lying on your back in a hospital bed. As your eyes begin to search your surroundings, that's when the pain hits you—a searing ache in your skull, as if giant apes were playing volleyball with your noggin. "You took quite a knock to your head, there," says a nurse standing nearby looking over your chart. You stare at her blankly. "You don't remember?" she continues. You shake your head, no. "Your friend hit you in the head with a baseball bat by accident," the nurse says matter-of-factly. All you can do is groan at this bit of news. "That's okay, take your time," the nurse says gently.

You close your eyes again, but the pain is still intense. A doctor traipses in. "Ah, you're awake," he says cheerily, "that's good." He takes out one of those little pocket flashlights doctors use to check your eyes, and shines it smack in your face. "Mmmm . . . hmmmm . . .

looks good," he mumbles. "So," he continues, "can you talk? What's your name? Can you tell me who the president is?"

Of course I remember my goddamn name! you say to yourself. You say your name out loud, but it sounds bizarre—as if your own lips mouthed the words but another voice spoke them. "That's weird!" you think. Next you say the president's name. Same thing. You know you're pronouncing the word "Obama" as you always have, but when you say it now it's coming out sounding like you're a prim and proper BBC news anchor. You look up at the doctor, who seems puzzled as well. Although your chart says you're from Reading, Pennsylvania, you sound like you just got off the boat from Reading, England. What the hell, indeed!

You're suffering from a brain disorder called foreign accent syndrome—or FAS, for short. Foreign accent syndrome is *not* what made Madonna suddenly speak in plummy English tones when she married Guy Ritchie and moved to London (that's called pretentiousness!). FAS is an actual recognized medical condition.

WHAT IS IT?

FAS is a neurological disorder in which out of the blue a person begins to speak in an accent entirely different from the one they've always had.

ORIGINS

The first documented case of FAS was described by the highly regarded French neurologist Pierre Marie in 1907. Marie's study concerned a Parisian man who began to speak with the accent of an inhabitant of the Alsace region of France. Another early case study was by the famed German neurologist and psychologist Arnold Pick, who in 1919 described a Czech woman who started to speak with a Polish accent.

But the most thorough early study of FAS was by the Norwegian neurologist Georg Herman (G. H.) Monrad-Krohn. In 1947, Monrad-Krohn reported on the strange case of a Norwegian woman who'd been struck in the head by shrapnel during a 1941 German air raid over Oslo. The woman, known as Astrid L., suffered temporary paralysis, seizures, and severe speech impairment. Over time, her speech improved, but, as it did, her voice took on what sounded like a German accent—although she'd never traveled outside of Norway. As post-war Norwegians had no happy memories of their occupation by the Nazis, Astrid's new accent incited suspicions from some of her countrymen that she was a German collaborator.

Since these early days, about sixty cases of FAS have been reported worldwide. However, many researchers suspect that the number of cases is much higher, as FAS sufferers may not come forward due to embarrassment or the belief that nothing is really wrong with them—other than that they now "sound funny."

WHAT CAUSES IT?

What causes FAS? In short, nobody knows for sure; or, at least nothing is certain about the cause. Other than that, in the large majority of cases, it occurs after a brain injury, stroke, or similar type of neurological damage, such as a brain hemorrhage or multiple sclerosis. But why an injury to the brain causes a person to speak in an entirely different accent remains a medical mystery.

Some researchers have suspected FAS is caused by damage to a portion of the left hemisphere of the brain that's responsible for linguistic function. Studies have shown that some patients with FAS have lesions or other damage in these parts of the brain. Thus, researchers surmise damage to this area results in changes to a person's pronunciation, as well as the tone and timbre of his or her voice.

Yet, another theory says damage to the brain's neural circuits isn't solely responsible. For this second group, FAS is most likely a result of post-injury changes in a patient's speech patterns. The complex intersection of neural circuits and fine motor skills required to produce sounds is out of whack, and the patient sounds "different" than he or she used to sound.

A third possibility suggests genetics could be a factor in a small number of cases. Researchers in Belgium studied patients with FAS who had no previous brain injury, nor any lesions in the brain area known to affect language. In these cases, a genetic mutation is one possible cause for the appearance of FAS.

> **The Upside of...**
> **Foreign Accent**
> **Syndrome**
>
> - It's a whole new you without spending any money on clothes or plastic surgery.
> - Offer yourself up for foreign roles at local theater companies.
> - The perfect reason to finally move abroad.

One factor that scientists have absolutely ruled out as a cause of FAS is that it's a psychological problem. Many FAS sufferers confront disbelief from family, friends, and even doctors about the change in their accent. But FAS is not a "put-on," a la Madonna; it is real, and patients have no control over the sound of their voice.

SIGNS AND SYMPTOMS

After a head injury, stroke, or similar event, FAS sufferers will speak in an accent different from the one they had before their injury. The patient may now elongate syllables, mispronounce words in a way typical of a foreign speaker of his or native language, or the rhythm of his or her voice may be altered. However, one very interesting fact about FAS is that the accent can be mutable—one day a person with FAS might sound Swedish; the next day the same patient might sound more German or Italian.

DIAGNOSIS AND TREATMENT

Symptoms may last months or years, but many sufferers respond well to speech therapy. Counseling may also be necessary as many patients report feeling a profound loss of identity due to the change in their voice.

PROGNOSIS

With therapy, symptoms can be relieved.

PREVALENCE

FAS is very rare and researchers are unsure of how many cases there are.

HOW TO AVOID IT

Other than not being whacked upside the head by a bat or other blunt object, you should take all the precautions you can to avoid a stroke, as strokes are the most common cause of FAS. This means eating right, exercising, and keeping a close watch on your blood pressure.

NOTABLE CASES

Since the historical cases noted above, a few other high-profile occurrences of FAS have caught researchers—and the media's—attention:

- While recovering from a stroke in 1999, a fifty-seven-year-old Florida woman who'd previously had a New York accent began to speak with a British accent. Embarrassed by her condition, the woman avoided social contact and developed agoraphobia. Finally, in 2003, she was referred to researchers at the University of Central Florida, who helped diagnose and treat her case of FAS.

- In 2006, a sixty-year-old British woman from northeast England suffered a stroke. When she awakened in the hospital her typically northeastern accent now sounded Jamaican (although others described the accent as Eastern European).

- In 2007, a woman in Port Angeles, Washington, saw her chiropractor to have her back and neck adjusted. Following the appointment, her neck swelled up and three days later she started speaking in an accent variously described as Swedish, Russian, and German. A stroke ruled out, doctors figured she'd developed foreign accent syndrome as a result of the chiropractor agitating a brain injury from 1981—in that year, the woman had fallen out of a moving truck, resulting in a fractured skull.

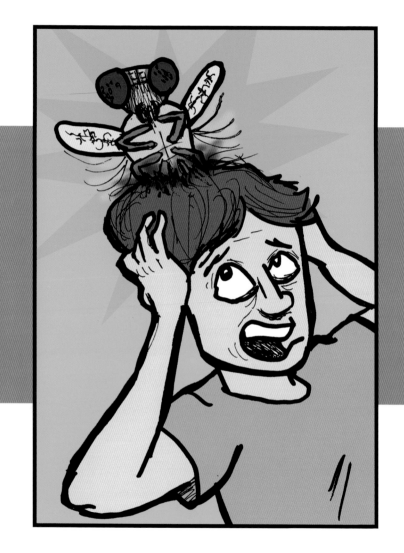

HUMAN BOTFLY MYIASIS

Ah, Costa Rica! Paradise found. The rain forest, the ocean, the wildlife! It was all so intoxicating. But now you're back home, and in addition to adjusting to the mundane workaday details of your life the past several weeks, you have a nagging pain on your back where you were bitten by a mosquito while on vacation. As the days go by, the former mosquito bite continues to grow into a boil-like bump; occasionally, pain shoots from the area and then subsides. Finally, you ask your friend to take a closer look at it and tell you what he sees. You lift the back of your shirt, and your friend peers closely at the bump, and then he shrieks, "It's alive!" *What the fuck does he mean, it's alive?* you think to yourself. "There is some goddamn thing alive *in* your back!" your friend continues. "There is some little white thing sticking out of your back, and it is freaking moving."

Looks like you brought home a "friend" from Costa Rica, in the form of a human botfly larva.

WHAT IS IT?

Human botfly myiasis occurs when humans are infected with the larvae of the fly species *Dermatobia hominis*. The larvae grow just below the skin and then emerge after six to ten weeks.

ORIGINS

Myiasis is Greek for "infestation of the body by the larvae of flies." No one knows how long human botfly myiasis has plagued mankind, but the Internet has certainly made it much more popular. Several amateur videos depict removal of the larvae from various body parts of affected individuals.

WHAT CAUSES IT?

It may not make you feel much better if you actually have botfly myiasis, but by generously lending your body as a home for its larvae, you're playing a vital role in the life cycle of the *Dermatobia hominis* fly. Here's what happens:

- ☒ Typically, a female botfly captures a mosquito in mid-air and deposits ten to fifty sticky eggs onto the mosquito's underside.
- ☒ Next the egg-laden mosquito finds you, pricks you, and proceeds to feed on your blood. When the mosquito finishes its meal, it flies away, but it leaves behind the tiny eggs, right next to the hole in your skin made by its proboscis.

☒ After about five minutes of incubating on your warm skin, each botfly egg hatches into a tiny larva. Using mouth hooks and tiny spines on its body, the larva wriggles into the opening of the mosquito bite.

☒ Beneath your skin the cozy larva feeds on your tissue, growing through two more larval stages in the course of six to ten weeks. Because it needs oxygen to grow, a very small piece of the white larva sticks out from the former mosquito bite wound so it can breathe.

☒ By the six- to ten-week mark, you'll know something is wrong with you and probably seek treatment. But if you're particularly out of it (or particularly gross), the next stage in the larval life cycle is that the now-one-inch-long larva pushes its way out of the skin. Ideally, the larva would like to land in some dirt into which it will burrow, and then, in four to eleven weeks, emerge as an adult botfly. Somewhat bizarrely, for all of the effort involved to reach maturity, the adult botfly only lives for a few days—which it spends mating and then, if female, laying eggs.

SIGNS AND SYMPTOMS

The first sign of a botfly infestation is a raised bump on the skin. Instead of getting better, this protuberance will grow over the course of several weeks. It may be painful when the larva shifts positions, and it also may be itchy. You also might see or feel the larva moving, particularly when you bathe or when the larva is covered. Because the wound remains open so the larva has oxygen, it will leak pus as the body sends white blood cells to try to heal itself.

DIAGNOSIS AND TREATMENT

A diagnosis of human botfly myiasis is made if you have the above symptoms and have traveled to a location known to have human botflies.

Treatment of human botfly myiasis involves removal of the larva from below the skin. One popular technique is to cut off the little bugger's oxygen supply by covering the wound with petroleum jelly, beeswax, bacon fat, duct tape, or even chewing gum. The botfly larva then pokes its head out of the wound to breathe, at which point it can be removed with a forceps. A second method is to inject the wound with anesthetic and cut the larva out. Sometimes the larva can simply be squeezed out. Yet another treatment technique is to do nothing at all, and let nature take its course.

The Upside of...
Human Botfly Myiasis

- Become an instant YouTube celebrity.
- The ultimate test of true love: "Honey, will you help me remove this fly larva that's popping out of my skin?"
- Have a pretty good shot at winning a "grossest thing that's ever happened to you" contest among your friends (unless a friend happens to have had Guinea worm disease).

After removal of the larva, antibiotics are usually prescribed to prevent infection.

PROGNOSIS

Amazingly, for something so gross, human botfly myiasis is generally not a serious problem. In rare cases, the larva can grow in body cavities such as the eyes, ears, or nose—and there are also documented cases of larva being lodged in the genital areas. These cases are more serious, and removal of the larva can be a complicated, and risky, procedure that requires skilled medical attention.

PREVALENCE

The *Dermatobia hominis* fly is found in parts of Mexico and in Central and South America. Despite alarms raised on the Internet, human botfly infections are relatively rare occurrences. There are no exact figures regarding the number of infections, but, suffice to say, thousands of people visit countries with human botflies every year without ever becoming infected.

HOW TO AVOID IT

If you travel to an area where the human botfly lives, at least wear mosquito repellant. Your best bet to avoid an infestation is to cover up as much of your body as is practical, and sleep with a mosquito net around your bed.

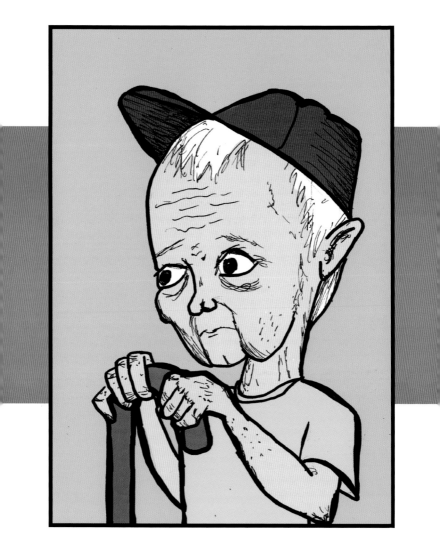

HUTCHINSON-GILFORD PROGERIA SYNDROME

Probably since the first human saw his or her reflection in a pond and noticed a gray hair, people have been trying to defy the aging process. Billions of dollars a year are spent on "miracle" potions, creams, pills, and fancy exercise gizmos that claim to make you look and feel younger (Bowflex, anyone?). But, what if instead of complaining about your aching back at age forty, you were grousing about it at age four? And what if thinning hair, wrinkly skin, and heart disease weren't worries you faced starting in middle age, but issues you confronted in primary school? Sound like a nightmare? Well, these tormented scenarios are just the kind of thing that kids—yes, kids!—with Hutchinson-Gilford progeria syndrome (or just progeria, for short) must deal with every day.

> ☝ **The Upside of...**
> **Progeria**
>
> - Probably the saddest known disease on earth.
> - No, really, there's nothing funny about this.
> - After reading this chapter, you will want to cry . . . .

WHAT IS IT?

Progeria is a rare genetic condition that causes accelerated aging of the body in children. Progeria is a fatal condition with no known cure.

ORIGINS

The name *progeria* is Greek for "prematurely old." Progeria was first described in 1886 by the English doctor Jonathan Hutchinson. The following year another Englishman, Hastings Gilford, described the condition further. The two docs were rewarded for their efforts by having the disorder named after them.

WHAT CAUSES IT?

For more than a hundred years, no one had any concrete insight into the causes of progeria. Then, in 2003, researchers identified the gene responsible for the condition: the LMNA gene. This gene encodes a protein that is an essential part of the membrane around cell nuclei. What researchers believe is that the mutated LMNA gene causes cell nuclei to become unstable, and this cell instability leads to premature aging.

SIGNS AND SYMPTOMS

Children born with progeria appear healthy at birth, but begin to display the first signs of the disorder at eighteen to twenty-four months. Symptoms include:

- ☒ Stunted growth
- ☒ Pinched, shrunken face
- ☒ Hair loss
- ☒ Wrinkled skin
- ☒ Loss of body fat
- ☒ Stiff joints
- ☒ Atherosclerosis
- ☒ Heart disease
- ☒ Respiratory problems
- ☒ Stroke

Of note is that, while the body grows old at a rapid rate, the mind is unaffected. Children with progeria are of normal intelligence and their cognitive development is the same as their peers.

DIAGNOSIS AND TREATMENT

Progeria is diagnosed through analyzing the signs and symptoms displayed by the child.

Sadly there is no cure for progeria. Treatments consist of attempting to minimize its negative effects, and include:

- ☒ Heart bypass surgery for blocked arteries
- ☒ Low-dose aspirin to help prevent heart attack and stroke
- ☒ High-calorie nutritional supplements to help prevent weight loss and provide necessary nutrients
- ☒ Physical and occupational therapy to help kids remain active

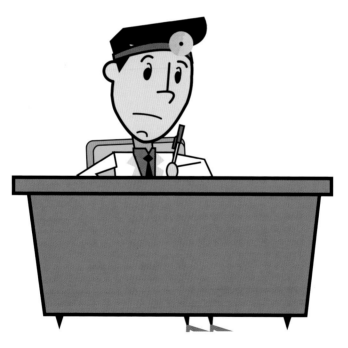

PROGNOSIS

Children with progeria generally live between eight and twenty-one years; the average life expectancy is thirteen years. Heart disease is the most common cause of death.

PREVALENCE

One in four to eight million children is born with progeria. It affects both sexes and all races equally. According to the Progeria Research Foundation, in 2006, there were forty-two children living in twenty different countries who'd been diagnosed with progeria.

HOW TO AVOID IT

Although progeria is a genetic disease, it is not passed down from parent to child. Indeed, children with the disease rarely live to childbearing age. The genetic mutation of the LMNA gene that causes progeria is a chance occurrence. Thus, there is no way to avoid getting the disorder.

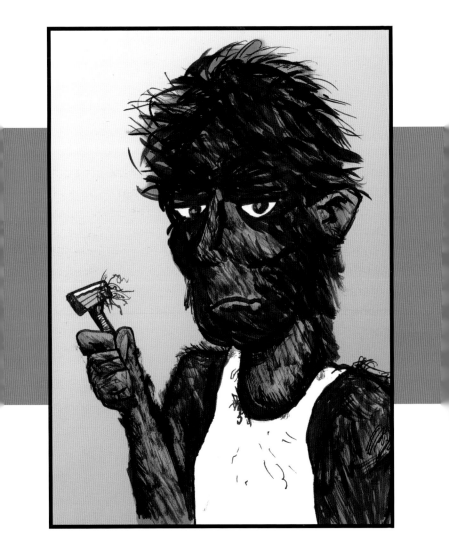

HYPERTRICHOSIS (HUMAN WEREWOLF SYNDROME)

"Dog-boy," "ape-man," "werewolf" . . . These are some of the inglorious names used through the centuries to describe sufferers of hypertrichosis, a condition characterized by excessive body hair growth. You may have heard of Jo Jo the Dog-Faced Boy or Lionel the Lion-Faced Man. These are two of the more infamous sufferers of this rare disorder, men who became renowned as sideshow freaks and performers.

WHAT IS IT?

Hypertrichosis is a general medical term that simply means hair growth beyond what is considered normal for a person's age, race, and sex. The hair may be exceedingly long or coarse, or it may look and feel like typical hair, yet grow abundantly in places where hair is usually thinner— or even typically nonexistent. Hair growth also may be local—occurring only on certain parts of the body, such as the chest, back, or arms—or it may be general, covering virtually the entire body.

ORIGINS

Hypertrichosis has no doubt been around for thousands of years, although the first documented case was that of Pedro Gonzales in the sixteenth century (see below).

WHAT CAUSES IT?

Before we discuss what might turn you into Teen Wolf, it helps to have some idea of the different kinds of human hair (yes, there are distinct varieties of hair). First, there are lanugo hairs—the long silky hairs that develop on a fetus while it's still in utero and that are normally shed before birth. Next are vellus hairs, which grow after the lanugo hairs are shed. Vellus hair is the short non-pigmented peach fuzz that covers an infant's whole body, except for the scalp and eyebrows. Finally, there's terminal hair, the coarser and colored hair that covers the scalp and eyebrows, and later, during puberty, grows on the arms and legs, groin, and underarms.

That rundown of the types of human hair is significant because just as there are different sorts of hair, there also are different varieties of hypertrichosis.

> **The Upside of... Hypertrichosis**
>
> - The cultural obsession with vampires must wear out eventually, and you know that werewolves are next!
> - Never have to buy a Halloween costume ever again.
> - Save money on shaving products.

- **Generalized Hypertrichosis**

This is the most dramatic form of hypertrichosis, in which the entire body, save for the palms of the hands and the soles of the feet, is covered in hair. In most cases of generalized hypertrichosis, the hair is lanugo hair that was never shed. However, in Ambras syndrome—a variety of generalized congenital hypertrichosis—the hairs are thick and coarse, and the amount of hair tends to increase with age.

It is thought that generalized congenital hypertrichosis is a result of an extremely rare genetic mutation. Only 100 cases have ever been documented worldwide.

- **Localized Hypertrichosis**

When excessive hair grows in patches, it is considered localized hypertrichosis. This condition may occur due to inborn genetic issues, or it can occur because of damage to the skin, underlying medical problems, or from certain drugs.

SIGNS AND SYMPTOMS

The defining symptom is hair—and a lot of it—where it should not be, or where it is not typically found in such great quantity.

DIAGNOSIS AND TREATMENT

Diagnosis of hypertrichosis first involves ruling out any other conditions that could cause excessive hair growth. Doctors will usually ask about the history of hair growth in one's family, and about drug use, such as if you're taking steroids. Women may have a blood test to check their hormone levels.

Once a diagnosis of hypertrichosis is established, treatment takes a few forms. One form of treatment is to do nothing about it, and live hairy. For those bothered by their excess hair, it may be removed by various methods, including electrolysis, laser removal, and intense pulsed light (IPL) treatments.

PROGNOSIS

Hypertrichosis cases caused by taking certain medications, or that result from other medical problems, will go away when the underlying issues are addressed. In cases where there are no underlying issues, you're stuck with the hair.

PREVALENCE

Generalized hypertrichosis is extremely rare. About 50 to 100 cases have been documented in medical literature since the Middle Ages. Figures on the number of cases of localized hypertrichosis are not available, but it is certainly more common than the generalized variety.

HOW TO AVOID IT

If you're genetically predisposed to hypertrichosis, there's not much you can do to avoid it. However, the condition also can develop as a reaction to certain drugs. The drugs most often indicated as causing hypertrichosis include: acetazolamide,corticosteroids, cyclosporin, danazol, diazoxide, hexachlorobenzene, minoxidil, penicillamine, psoralens, streptomycin, and tricyclic antidepressants.

NOTABLE CASES

▪ **Pedro Gonzalez**

The first documented case of generalized hypertrichosis was that of Pedro (or Petrus) Gonzalez. Born in the Canary Islands around 1537 (his exact birth date was never known), Gonzales was covered entirely with long silky lanugo hair. Regarded as some freakish human/animal hybrid by his contemporaries, Gonzales was sent to France as a gift to the court of King Henry II and his wife, Catherine de' Medici. In France it was quickly discovered that Gonzales was a perfectly normal human, who simply was much hairier than the average man. He was educated in literature, learned several languages, and eventually married. He and his wife had several children, most of whom also had hypertrichosis (though not all the offspring were hairy). The Gonzales family eventually settled in Italy, where Gonzales lived out his life.

Gonzales's form of generalized hypertrichosis was later named Ambras syndrome, after the famed Ambras Castle near Innsbruck, Austria. The castle houses a gallery called the Chamber of Art and Curiosities, a stunning collection of art devoted to human curiosities of the Renaissance era. A painting of Gonzales in the collection led to his condition being termed Ambras syndrome.

- Fedor Jeftichew

Born in 1868 in St. Petersburg, Russia, Jeftichew suffered from generalized hypertrichosis. His father also had the condition, and the two performed in circuses together. Following the elder Jeftichew's death, Fedor signed a contract with P. T. Barnum and arrived in the United States in 1884. Renamed Jo Jo the Dog-Faced Boy, Jeftichew performed with Barnum's circus throughout the U.S. and Europe. Jeftichew died in January 1904 of pneumonia.

- **Stephan Bibrowski**

Another of Barnum's circus freak acts, Bibrowski was born in Poland in 1891. His mother believed his condition was the result of his father being mauled by a lion while she was pregnant with Stephan. His mother gave him up to a German show business impresario when Stephan was four. The impresario, known as Meyer, renamed him Lionel the Lion-Faced Man. In 1901 Lionel traveled to the U.S. and began to tour in Barnum's circus, in which he performed gymnastics tricks and spoke to the audience, to show off his supposed gentle side. In truth, Bibrowski was highly educated and spoke five languages. In 1920 he settled in New York and became a popular performer at Coney Island for several years. By the late 1920s, he retired from performing and returned to Germany. He is said to have died of a heart attack in Berlin in 1932.

- **Jesús "Chuy" Aceves**

Aceves is the modern equivalent of Barnum's circus freaks. Born in Mexico, he is the second person in his family to have generalized hypertrichosis (his sister, a police officer, also has it). As a child, Aceves and his sister were displayed as medical wonders. Later, he performed in circuses as the Wolf Boy. Today, Aceves is in his mid-thirties and works backstage in the circus and occasionally performs in freak shows.

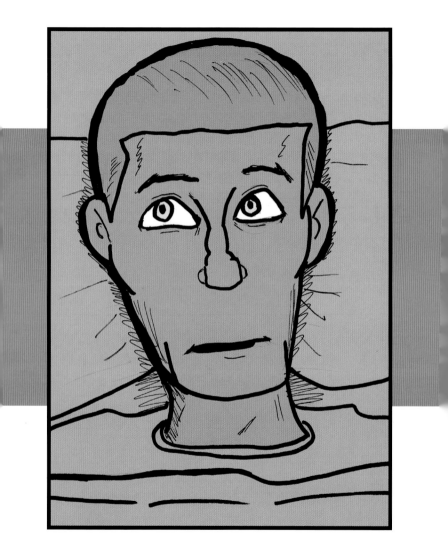

LOCKED-IN SYNDROME

You awaken in a hospital bed. You cannot move. You try to turn your head, but it's impossible. You try to speak to the nurse in the room, but no sound comes out. "It's a miracle you're alive," the nurse says. You want to say, "Thanks," but again nothing comes out. A slow, terrible realization washes over you: It is impossible for you to move anything but your eyes.

WHAT IS IT?

Locked-in syndrome is a rare neurological condition in which a patient remains completely conscious and mentally aware, yet is unable to move any part of his or her body, except for the eyes. It has been described as having your mind buried alive in a dead body.

ORIGINS

The name locked-in syndrome was coined by doctors Jerome Posner and Fred Plum in their landmark 1966 study, "Diagnosis of Stupor and Coma."

WHAT CAUSES IT?

Locked-in syndrome is caused by damage to the lower brain and brain stem, the areas that control voluntary muscle movement, while the upper brain remains unaffected. It may be caused by a stroke, trauma to the brain from injury, a brain hemorrhage, diseases of the circulatory system, or an overdose of medication.

The Upside of...
Locked-In Syndrome

- Concrete proof that there really is a fate worse than death.
- Pretty much the most awful thing you could think of.
- Not . . . good . . .

SIGNS AND SYMPTOMS

Complete paralysis, except for movement of the eyes.

DIAGNOSIS AND TREATMENT

No treatment exists for locked-in syndrome. Some patients have learned to communicate by a system of blinking in code.

PROGNOSIS

Motor function usually does not return at all. In 90 percent of cases, patients with locked-in syndrome die within four months of the condition's onset.

PREVALENCE

It isn't known how many locked-in syndrome cases there are.

HOW TO AVOID IT

Many of the causes of locked-in syndrome are out of your control. To minimize the ones you do have control over—stroke and medicine overdose, for example—do all you can to maintain your health.

NOTABLE CASES

▪ **Jean-Dominique Bauby**

In 1995 the French editor of *Elle* magazine, Jean-Dominique Bauby, suffered a stroke. When he awoke from a coma twenty days later, he was unable to move any part of his body, except for his left eyelid. Bauby developed a complicated method of communication by blinking his eyelid. Painstakingly, he was able to dictate his memoir, *The Diving Bell and the Butterfly*, letter by letter. He died of pneumonia two days after the book was published in March 1997.

▪ **Erik Ramsey**

After a car accident in 1999, sixteen-year-old Erik Ramsey suffered a stroke that resulted in locked-in syndrome. Today, the Georgia man is working with researchers to see if they can translate the neurological activity in his brain when he thinks of words into sounds through a computer.

▪ **Julia Tavalaro**

In 1966, at age thirty-two, Tavalaro suffered two strokes and a brain hemorrhage. Doctors thought she was in a vegetative state, but six years after her stroke a family member thought Tavalaro tried to smile after hearing a joke. A speech therapist recognized in Tavalaro's eye movements that she could hear and understand when someone spoke to her. Tavalaro learned to blink in code to communicate and went on to become a poet and writer. She died in 2003 at age sixty-eight.

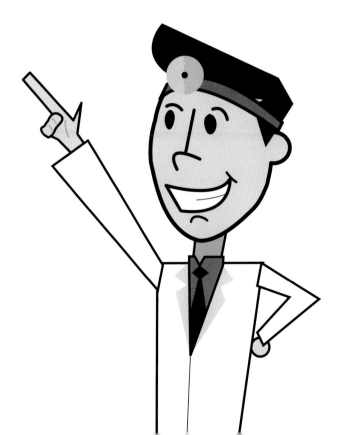

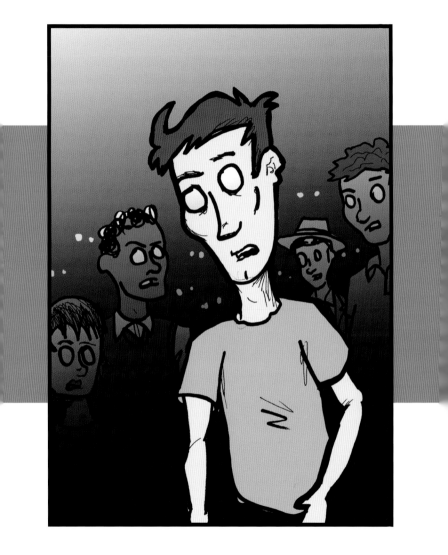

MASS PSYCHOGENIC ILLNESS

It all started innocently enough. There was a smell wafting through your office—a weird bleach-like smell. At first no one thought much of it. "Probably cleaning the carpets on four again," said one co-worker, which seemed the most logical explanation. But after a couple of days, the smell hadn't dissipated. Then, at lunch, another colleague excitedly asked you, "Did you hear that Rick from accounting got a terrible headache and got so dizzy that he nearly fainted?" You hadn't heard that. By 4 PM that same day, word had gotten around that five more people had left work after experiencing similar symptoms to Rick in accounting. By the end of the next day, half the office was complaining of headaches and dizziness. Could it be carbon monoxide poisoning? The day after that, three-quarters of your co-workers called in sick. But Rick in accounting was back in the office. He'd been to the doctor and had a physical exam and tests said he was perfectly healthy. What's more, your company called in a firm to analyze the air in the office, and those tests revealed nothing abnormal in the air. So what was making everybody so sick?

The answer, of course, is that their own minds were making them sick. This is a classic case of mass psychogenic illness.

WHAT IS IT?

Mass psychogenic illness is a sociopsychological phenomenon that occurs when a large group of people exhibits signs of being sick, despite the fact that there are no physical or environmental factors present that would make them ill.

ORIGINS

Outbreaks of mass psychogenic illness have been happening for centuries. Probably ever since humans starting living in groups, we've been susceptible to such episodes of mass hysteria. But some of the earliest recorded instances of mass psychogenic illness date to medieval times (see "Notable Cases" below).

WHAT CAUSES IT?

Episodes of mass psychogenic illness begin with a trigger. The trigger may be a smell, a sound, or even a thought that's passed along from person to person. These triggers cause stress in the surrounding population and that stress can have a powerful effect on people's emotions and behavior. The strong belief that one may get sick is only reinforced by the knowledge that others are sick around you. Media coverage of outbreaks, or seeing ambulances or emergency workers, only heightens stress levels, giving people even more reason to think they might be ill too. Perfectly healthy, otherwise socially well-adjusted people are as likely as anyone else to fall prey to mass psychogenic illness.

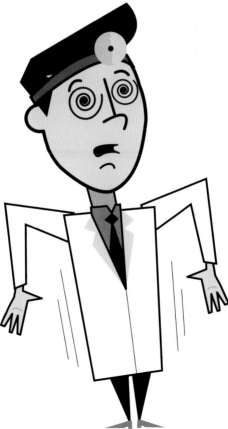

SIGNS AND SYMPTOMS

The symptoms of mass psychogenic illness depend on the type of hysteria being experienced. But the most common symptoms people experience are:

- ☒ Headache
- ☒ Dizziness
- ☒ Nausea
- ☒ Fainting
- ☒ Weakness

It should be noted that while there are no physical or environmental causes for the above symptoms, the symptoms are real. In other words, people really do get headaches, they really do feel dizzy, and they really can faint. They aren't faking their symptoms. However, these responses are psychosomatic—the result of stress, not actual illness.

DIAGNOSIS AND TREATMENT

Mass psychogenic illness is suspected when there's no discernible cause for the problems people are having.

Treatment of mass psychogenic illness is complicated, of course, by the fact that there is no actual illness to treat. Thus, most of the tactics involved in stopping an outbreak involve managing the stress and anxiety around the situation. The following steps are usually taken to help bring the hysteria to a halt:

- ☒ Separation of the affected people from the environment that caused their symptoms. Most patients recover quickly once they're away from where they acquired the symptoms.
- ☒ Physical exams and tests of affected individuals
- ☒ Acknowledgement that patients are experiencing real symptoms, but that no cause has been found for their ailments
- ☒ Explanations of how stress and anxiety can affect people individually and as a group

PROGNOSIS

If the treatment guidelines above are followed, episodes of mass psychogenic illness end relatively quickly and everyone involved is able to return to their normal lives.

The Upside of...
Mass Psychogenic Illness

- Yes, you really are just another member of the herd.
- Convenient excuse for teens attending an all-night dance party: "But, Mom, I was a victim of mass psychogenic illness!"
- Proof you don't need fancy gadgets to really fuck with people.

PREVALENCE

No official body tracks outbreaks of mass psychogenic illness. Episodes are liable to occur in any culture throughout the world, and may affect any strata of society.

HOW TO AVOID IT

Live as a hermit, avoiding contact with any large groups of people.

NOTABLE CASES

▪ **Dancing Plague of 1518**

One of the first documented cases of mass psychogenic illness is the dancing plague that struck Strasbourg, France, in July of 1518. It began when a woman started dancing in the street for no apparent reason, and then continued to dance for several days. She was joined at first by a few other townspeople, yet within a month some 400 Strasbourgers were dancing maniacally in the open air. By the time the so-called plague was over, dozens of the dancers had died from exhaustion, heart attacks, and strokes.

Scientists today believe the plague was brought on by stress and anxiety. Preceding the dancing mania, the region around Strasbourg had been hit by a famine that killed many people. In addition, weakened by the famine, many fell prey to diseases such as leprosy, smallpox, and syphilis. The craze may have been further spurred on by a legend associated with St. Vitus, the patron saint of dancing. That said, if Vitus was angered, he would cause people to dance uncontrollably.

▪ Tanganyika Laughter Epidemic

In 1962 the East African territory of Tanganyika (now a part of Tanzania) fell prey to one of the weirdest epidemics of all time: uncontrollable laughing. The laughter started with a group of schoolgirls and spread throughout the area, affecting thousands of people. Schools were shut down, and the epidemic took six to eighteen months to fully die down. In addition to laughing, people complained of fainting, crying, rashes, and respiratory problems.

▪ Perfume "Sickens" Texans

In July 2009, nearly 150 workers were sickened at a Bank of America call center in Fort Worth, Texas. Thirty-four workers were taken to hospitals complaining of dizziness and shortness of breath. Emergency workers at first thought the employees might be suffering from carbon monoxide poisoning, but an investigation found that it was someone's perfume odor that set off the whole event.

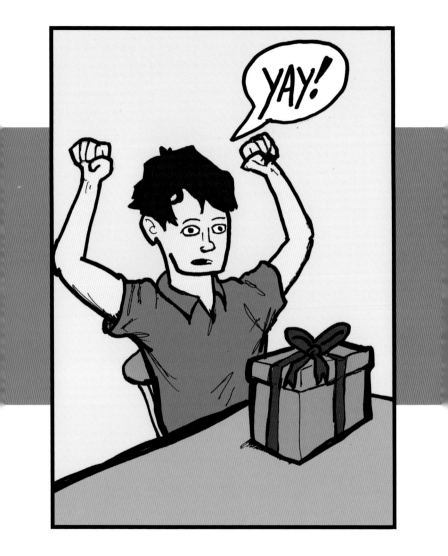

MOEBIUS SYNDROME

"For news of the heart, ask the face," goes a famous proverb. But what if you looked into someone's face and it offered no news at all? Not of the heart, nor about any other organ. And what if instead of offering a window into the soul, the eyes looked at you blankly, betraying no sense of their owner's innermost thoughts and emotions? But this person whose face you're gazing upon isn't some mime, nor is he or she trying to trick you by purposely maintaining a frozen visage. The face in front of you is expressionless because its owner *can't move it*!

WHAT IS IT?

Moebius syndrome is a congenital neurological disorder that results in complete facial paralysis. Sufferers are unable to close their eyes, and cannot make facial expressions; they're also unable to move their eyes laterally (i.e., in a back and forth motion).

ORIGINS

Moebius syndrome is named for the German neurologist Paul Julius Möbius, who was the first to describe it in 1884.

WHAT CAUSES IT?

Moebius syndrome is caused by underdevelopment, or the complete absence of, the sixth and seventh cranial nerves. These nerves, which directly come out of the brain stem, control one's facial expressions and eye movements. The reason these nerves are damaged is not clear. Most Moebius cases appear in families with no previous history of the syndrome. But researchers are still exploring possible genetic connections.

The Upside of...
Moebius Syndrome

- Beat your kid at staring contests—every time.
- Career as a poker player a definite good choice.
- Botox treatments never necessary.

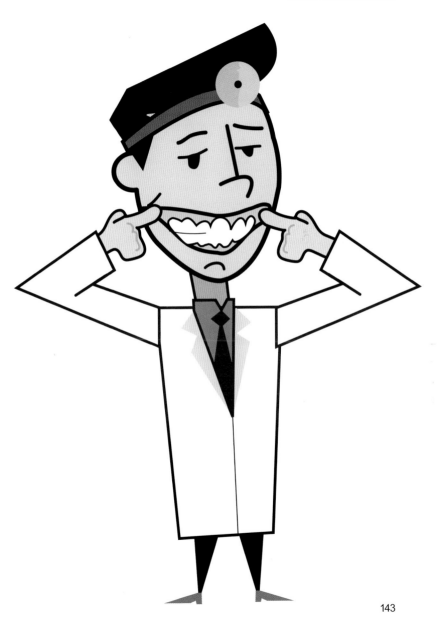

SIGNS AND SYMPTOMS

The first sign of Moebius syndrome is that a baby is unable to suck. Other symptoms include:

- ☒ Absence of blinking
- ☒ Lack of facial expressions
- ☒ Excessive drooling
- ☒ Crossed eyes
- ☒ Difficulty chewing and swallowing
- ☒ Cleft palate
- ☒ Short or deformed tongue
- ☒ Impaired motor development due to upper body weakness

DIAGNOSIS AND TREATMENT

A diagnosis of Moebius syndrome is made based on the presentation of symptoms listed above. There is no cure for it, so all the treatments are focused on managing the condition. Infants may have to be fed with a special bottle or via a feeding tube. Physical, occupational, and speech therapies can improve patients' speaking and eating abilities as they get older. Eye drops can combat chronic dry eyes due to the inability to blink, while surgery can correct crossed eyes. One extreme treatment is so-called "smile surgery," in which nerves and muscles from the inner thigh are transplanted to the corners of the mouth so that a patient can form a smile. The surgery also helps improve chewing.

PROGNOSIS

About 30 to 40 percent of Moebius syndrome patients suffer some degree of autism. But the majority of patients have normal mental capacity and live an average lifespan.

PREVALENCE

Moebius is a rare disorder and no one is certain how many people have it. The Moebius Syndrome Foundation—which was founded in 1994 to support patients and promote research—says it knows of roughly 2,000 people worldwide with the disorder.

The syndrome affects boys and girls equally.

HOW TO AVOID IT

As Moebius syndrome is a congenital disorder that is present at birth, there is nothing one can do to prevent getting it.

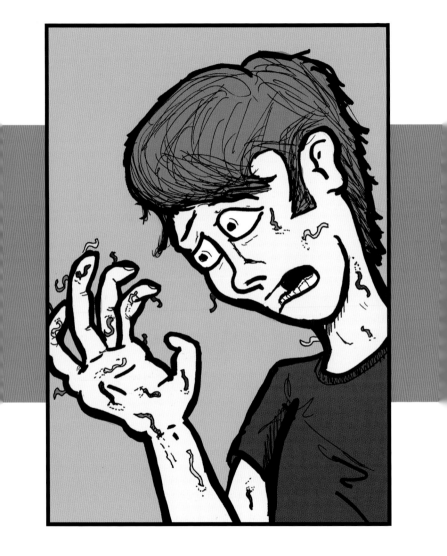

MORGELLONS DISEASE

For days, you've had the incredibly annoying sensation that bugs are crawling on and under your skin. You're well aware that this is a side effect of taking PCP, but you're no angel dust sniffer. Really, you aren't. You're just a regular normal person, with normal person worries and normal person problems—usually, at least. But this bug thing is truly freaking weird!

You don't want to seem nuts, so you've kept your ailment to yourself. But now, to go along with the invisible creepy crawlies torturing you, you've also developed sores on your skin—painful, ugly sores that itch like the dickens. And now things are getting even weirder: the sores have tiny little fibers coming out of them, like little colored hairs in red, black, white, and blue. Are you becoming an alien? You have no choice; you must go to the doctor.

The doctor examines your skin, looks puzzled, and then asks if you have any other symptoms—perhaps muscle pain, or trouble with your short-term memory? Yes, you have both of those problems, now that you think about it. The doctor nods and says, "I'm afraid it looks like you have Morgellons disease."

WHAT IS IT?

Morgellons is a poorly understood skin disorder that causes patients to feel crawling or biting sensations on or under the skin. It is also characterized by spontaneously erupting lesions (sores or rashes) that have filamentous fibers coming out of them.

ORIGINS

The name Morgellons disease was coined by a Pennsylvania mom, Mary Leitao, in 2002. Leitao, a former medical researcher and now executive director of the Morgellons Research Foundation, sought answers when her two-year-old son developed a strange rash under his lip, and started pointing to the rash and saying, "Bugs." Visits to several dermatologists yielded no cures and no explanation for the rash. Frustrated and angry, Leitao took it upon herself to start researching what could be plaguing her son.

During her investigation, Leitao came across a description from 1674 of a condition that afflicted children in the Languedoc region of France. As described by the

---

The Upside of...
Morgellons Disease

- Convenient excuse to take PCP. Shit, you've already got some of the effects; might as well just go whole hog!
- Spontaneously erupting lesions!
- Give new meaning to the phrase, "You're really bugging me."

---

famed English physician Sir Thomas Browne, the French kids had hairs growing on their backs. Browne referred to the phenomenon as "the Morgellons." As this description sounded similar to her son's condition, Leitao adopted the name Morgellons.

It is not clear that the condition described by Browne as Morgellons is at all the same as the modern illness. Indeed, Leitao simply borrowed the Morgellons tag because no other medical term fit the problem.

WHAT CAUSES IT?

There is no known cause of Morgellons disease. In fact, the disease is controversial within the medical research community. Morgellons' official designation by the U.S. Centers for Disease Control and Prevention (CDC) is as an "unexplained dermopathy." In January 2008, the CDC launched an investigation of suspected Morgellons cases in Northern California with help from Kaiser Permanente's Northern California Division of Research and the Armed Forces Institute of Pathology. But the CDC is withholding judgment for now about whether Morgellons is a real disorder or not.

Some doctors firmly believe research by the CDC and others will show that Morgellons is indeed a unique disorder. The Morgellons Research Foundation (a national organization devoted to furthering study of the condition) says on its Web site, "The cause is likely known bacteria missed by science because of incorrect early assumptions, much like Marshall's finding *Helicobacter pylori*, a common 'good' stomach parasite, turned out to be the primary cause of certain ulcers and gastritis . . . NOT stress and pizza."

Yet other researchers are convinced that Morgellons is not a disease unto itself. Those in the doubting camp point to the fact that many Morgellons symptoms are consistent with several other well-known conditions, including chronic fatigue syndrome, attention-deficit disorder, Lyme disease, and delusional parasitosis (in which a person believes his or her body is crawling with parasites).

SIGNS AND SYMPTOMS

- ☒ Painful and or itchy skin lesions
- ☒ Sensation of crawling, biting, or stinging on or under the skin
- ☒ Fibers growing out of or inside the lesions, usually colored white but also black, blue, and red
- ☒ Joint, muscle, and tendon pain (headaches and backaches are particularly common)
- ☒ Impaired vision
- ☒ Change in skin color and texture
- ☒ Intense fatigue
- ☒ Short-term memory loss, inability to concentrate or think clearly
- ☒ Depression

DIAGNOSIS AND TREATMENT

There is no known treatment for Morgellons. Several firms advertising online tout the alleged benefits of their "alternative remedies" for treating Morgellons symptoms. The CDC warns: "Consumers should seek input from their healthcare provider before purchasing or using any product (e.g., skin creams, pills, and other medications) or equipment that is marketed as a treatment for this condition."

PROGNOSIS

There is currently no cure for Morgellons.

PREVALENCE

Morgellons strikes both adults and children. It appears in isolated cases—where, for example, only one member of a family is affected—and in groups. Thus it's not known if the condition is inherited or contagious.

Incidences of Morgellons have been reported in every state in the U.S., with the most cases occurring in California, Texas, and Florida.

HOW TO AVOID IT

There doesn't appear to be any practical way to avoid getting Morgellons.

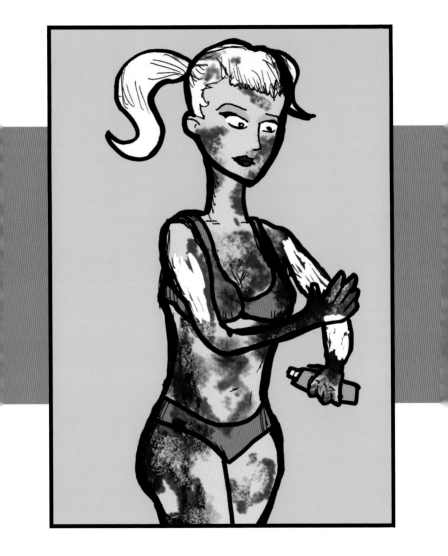

MUD WRESTLER'S RASH

The bachelor party is over. And while you can't remember much from two nights ago, the photos your best man just sent confirm that you did indeed jump shirtless into the mud-wrestling pit at Crazy Sam's Wild Cantina, to take on Tammy and Tina—the bar's very own pair of bikini-clad champion mud wrestlers. You can't remember if you beat the girls or they beat you, but either way you just hope your fiancée doesn't get a hold of the photographic evidence of the shenanigans. Well, either way you've gotta get up now and meet your parents, future in-laws, and your future wife for brunch. But damn, why do your arms itch like crazy?! You lift your arm to examine it, and—holy shit!—it's covered in little red bumps. What's more, the crazy rash is all over your chest too. This . . . is . . . not . . . good.

WHAT IS IT?

Mud wrestler's rash—or *dermatitis palaestrae limosae* ("dermatitis of muddy wrestling", in Latin)—is an unfortunate hazard of taking part in the classic American pastime.

ORIGINS

Mud wrestler's rash was first documented in a January 1993 article in the *Journal of the American Medical Association*. University of Washington student health center docs Amanda Adler and Jeff Altman are the lucky ones to have coined the name *dermatitis palaestrae limosae*, after examining collegiate mud wrestlers displaying the telltale rash.

WHAT CAUSES IT?

After an outbreak of the rash the day after a mud-wrestling event at the University of Washington in spring 1992, the two campus health center doctors tested pus taken from seven rash-ridden students. The doctors found fecal bacteria in the pus. Doctors then discovered similar fecal bacteria in the topsoil used to make the wrestling mud. Thus, the rash was a result of fecal bacteria in the mud penetrating the skin, most likely through hair follicles, or through cuts and abrasions. Interestingly, the rash was more prevalent among women wrestlers—which doctors ascribed to the fact that the bacteria more easily entered the hair follicles of the women's shaved legs.

SIGNS AND SYMPTOMS

Mud wrestler's rash manifests itself as itchy, red, pus-filled bumps that can appear on skin that's come into contact with mud from the wrestling ring. The rash usually appears twenty-four to thirty-six hours after exposure to the mud.

DIAGNOSIS AND TREATMENT

As with other skin irritations, medication successfully treats the rash.

PROGNOSIS

Left untreated, infection could occur. However, if treated promptly, those with mud wrestler's rash make a complete recovery.

PREVALENCE

Wherever there are drunk college students, you're likely to find cases of mud wrestler's rash. No reliable statistics exist as to the actual number of people affected each year.

👍 **The Upside of...**
Mud Wrestler's Rash

- Good luck explaining this one to your mate.
- It's a dirty and dangerous job, but someone's gotta take the risk.
- Grounds for the oddest workers' comp case in history.

HOW TO AVOID IT

If you must mud wrestle, be sure to use mud that has not been contaminated. Similarly, only hose down the mud with water that you're sure isn't contaminated.

NOTABLE CASES

At the 2009 Boryeong Mud Festival in South Korea, 200 revelers sought treatment after their skin erupted in a rash. The annual eight-day festival attracts more than a million people to roll around in mud trucked in and dumped on the banks of the Daecheon river. Ironically, the fest originated to publicize the quality of skin-care products made with the region's mineral-rich mud.

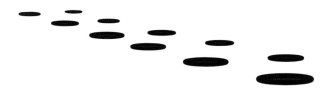

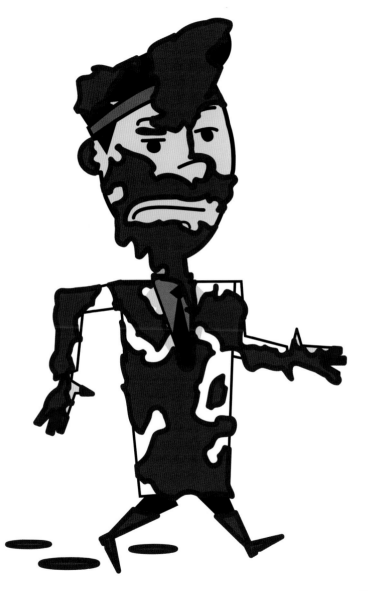

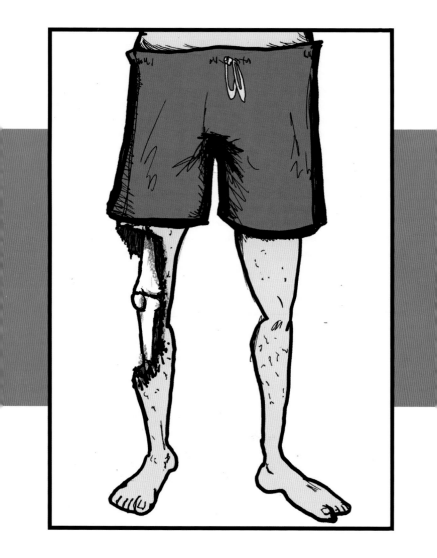

NECROTIZING FASCIITIS (FLESH-EATING BACTERIA)

It started with no apparent warning. Your leg just started to hurt. At first the pain wasn't bad, and you rubbed and rubbed your calf, trying to soothe the ache. There was nothing obviously wrong with your leg other than a tiny little cut you'd gotten a couple of days before. A few hours later, your lower leg started to swell. You felt feverish, nauseous, and weak. Could the flu come on this violently? You check on your leg again and it has turned a horrible shade of purple, and blisters are starting to form on the outside of the skin. What's more, your upper leg is now turning red, too. *What the fuck is going on?!* If you don't get to a hospital right away, you'll be dead in a few days.

WHAT IS IT?

Necrotizing fasciitis (NF) is a bacterial infection caused by several kinds of bacteria. The bacteria attack and destroy the soft tissues below the skin—fat and the fascia (fibrous tissue that connects and surrounds muscles). As the infection spreads it causes the body's organs to go into systemic shock, resulting in heart failure, respiratory failure, and renal failure. If left untreated, NF usually leads to death in a short time—anywhere from less than twenty-four hours to a few days.

ORIGINS

The first modern description of NF is credited to Joseph Jones, a Confederate Army surgeon in the Civil War. In describing several cases of what today appear to be NF, Jones called the affliction "hospital gangrene." Other names applied to the disease were necrotizing erysipelas, streptococcal gangrene, and suppurative fasciitis. The term necrotizing fasciitis was introduced in 1952.

WHAT CAUSES IT?

NF is caused by a variety of bacteria. The most common culprit is a bacterium called *Streptococcus pyogenes*, one of the Group A streptococcus (GAS) bacteria. Normally, GAS bacteria are fairly harmless, and can even be found living in the mouth and throat or on the skin of people who exhibit no symptoms of illness at all. Certain GAS strains are responsible for common infections like strep throat, scarlet fever, and impetigo. But in cases of NF, the GAS strains involved are very deadly.

In the majority of NF cases, the GAS bacteria enter the body through a break in the skin caused by a cut, scrape, burn, or surgical incision. Once inside the body, the bacteria reproduce and attack the soft tissues below the skin by giving off toxins and enzymes that kill the tissues.

While Group A streptococcus is the most common cause of NF, some other bacteria also are responsible: *Vibrio vulnificus*, *Staphylococcus aureus*, *Peptostreptococcus*, *Clostridium*, *Bacteroides*, *Klebsiella*, and *Proteus*.

One way NF is emphatically *not* transmitted is through Costa Rican bananas. In December 1999, an Internet hoax claimed that the monkey population in Costa Rica had been devastated by NF, and recommended that no one buy any bananas for three weeks. This was pure bullshit.

The Upside of...
Necrotizing Fasciitis

- And you thought flesh-eating bacteria wasn't real? Think again!
- Survive this and you'll have the best cocktail party story—ever.
- A horror film come to life—with you as the unwitting star.

SIGNS AND SYMPTOMS

Symptoms may be broken down into early symptoms that appear within the first twenty-four hours of infection and advanced symptoms that occur anywhere from a day to a few days after infection.

- **Early Symptoms**
  - ☒ Pain in the general area of a wound
  - ☒ The pain may be very great in proportion to the size of the injured area—the area around a small cut, for example, may hurt intensely
  - ☒ Swelling and redness of the skin
  - ☒ Flu-like symptoms: fever, nausea, vomiting, diarrhea, weakness, confusion
  - ☒ Dehydration

- **Advanced Symptoms**
  - ☒ Red skin may turn purplish and swelling continues
  - ☒ Fluid-filled blisters form on the skin
  - ☒ Skin may appear necrotic, turning a white or bluish hue and becoming flaky
  - ☒ Gangrene

DIAGNOSIS AND TREATMENT

Because early symptoms resemble those of many other conditions, NF is frequently misdiagnosed. A tissue biopsy can confirm the presence of bacteria that cause NF.

As you can imagine, treating NF is not a pretty picture.

The first thing you should do if you suspect you have NF is go to the hospital—immediately. At the hospital, you will be given intravenous antibiotics. Then a surgeon will be called. The only way to cure NF is to remove the affected tissue. This process is called "debridement." If you're really lucky, and you've caught the NF quickly and it hasn't spread too far, the surgeon will remove the gangrenous skin and tissue, and all you may be left with is some scarring. If you're unlucky, the doctor may have to amputate affected limbs.

In nearly every case, failure to treat NF will result in death in anywhere from eighteen hours to a few days, depending on the virulence of the infection and the type of bacteria involved.

PROGNOSIS

Chances for survival depend entirely on how quickly NF is treated. Roughly 20 to 30 percent of NF cases end in death.

PREVALENCE

According to the U.S. Centers for Disease Control and Prevention, there are about 500 to 800 cases of NF in the

U.S. per year. There is no higher incidence in any population based on age, race, or ethnic origin. But there are certain people with an increased likelihood of contracting NF. These include:

- ☒ People with weakened immune systems
- ☒ People with chronic health conditions, such as diabetes, cancer, or kidney and liver disease
- ☒ Children with chicken pox
- ☒ People taking medication that reduces immune system function (e.g., steroids or chemotherapy)

HOW TO AVOID IT

For obvious reasons, it's hard to prevent a bacterial infection. However, the good news is that you're very unlikely to get NF. Even if you come into contact with someone who has the infection, it's not usually contagious.

The best way to avoid getting NF is to use common-sense precautions: wash your hands frequently, and keep cuts, scrapes, burns, sores, bites, and other wounds clean and free of infection.

NOTABLE CASES

▪ **Jim Henson**

The Muppets creator died of toxic shock syndrome in 1990, after being infected by the *Streptococcus pyogenes* bacteria.

▪ **Lucien Bouchard**

Bouchard, a former premier of Québec and a leader of the Québec separatist movement, became infected in 1994. At first Bouchard thought he'd pulled a muscle in his leg. His leg was later amputated.

▪ **Eric Cornell**

Cornell, a research physicist and a Nobel Prize winner for physics in 2001, was infected with NF in October 2004. His left arm and shoulder were lost to the disease.

▪ **David Walton**

A prominent UK economist, Walton was a member of the Bank of England's Monetary Policy Committee when he contracted NF in June 2006. Doctors said he died within twenty-four hours of entering the hospital, despite extraordinary efforts to save him.

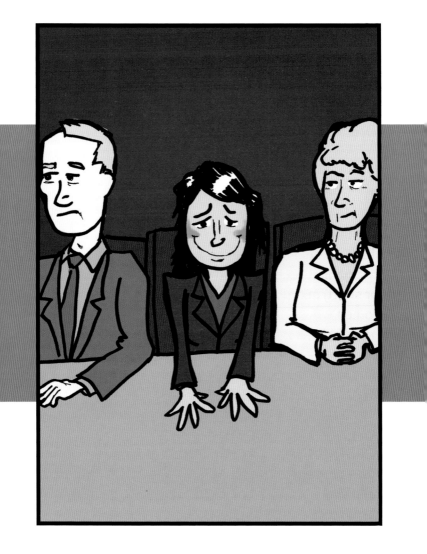

PERSISTENT SEXUAL AROUSAL SYNDROME/ PERSISTENT GENITAL AROUSAL DISORDER (PSAS/PGAD)

Just like with priapism in men (see chapter 28), at first blush persistent sexual arousal syndrome (or persistent genital arousal syndrome—or just PSAS/PGAD, for short) might seem pretty good. But for the rare few women who suffer from PSAS/PGAD, "suffer" is truly the right word.

Imagine sitting in a meeting at work when you suddenly become very, very aroused. Sure, charts and graphs of fourth-quarter growth estimates can be exciting, but that's not what has you hot and bothered. PSAS/PGAD appears without any sexual stimulation—physical or psychological. One moment you're making an important point to your colleagues, and the next you're squirming in your chair, your loins on fire. Not fun.

WHAT IS IT?

Women with persistent sexual arousal syndrome become genitally aroused for extended periods of time in the absence of any sexual stimulation or desire. Orgasms can be triggered by anything from the vibration of driving in a car to a touch from a friend, exercise, or simply walking.

ORIGINS

It's suspected that PSAS/PGAD is not new. But shame and embarrassment over its symptoms no doubt kept women from discussing it with doctors until recently.

PSAS/PGAD was first documented in a 2001 article, "Persistent Sexual Arousal Syndrome: A Newly Discovered Pattern of Female Sexuality" in the *Journal of Sex & Marital Therapy*. Co-authored by Dr. Sandra Leiblum—a noted sex therapist, researcher, and author based in New Jersey—and New York psychologist Dr. Sharon Nathan, the article detailed five cases of PSAS/PGAD in the hope that the authors' findings would stimulate (no pun intended) further research.

WHAT CAUSES IT?

Considering only a few researchers are studying PSAS/PGAD, it's no surprise that the condition is not very well understood. One thing is certain, though: it is *not* the same thing as hypersexuality, aka, nymphomania.

One theory is that PSAS/PGAD is a nervous system disorder. The problem could lie within the complex system of sensory nerves in the brain and spinal cord. Perhaps the nervous system is mistakenly stimulating the sexual organs.

Other possible causes include:

⊠ Pelvic surgery or trauma
⊠ Brain lesions
⊠ Hypersensitivity of nerves in the pelvis
⊠ Arteriovenous malformation (AVM) in the pelvis, a condition where there is an abnormal connection between the veins and arteries in the pelvic area
⊠ Side effect of stopping antidepressants
⊠ Psychological factors

The Upside of...
PSAS/PGAD

- Apparently, it really is possible to have too much of a good thing.
- The ultimate itch that can't be scratched.
- "Hold on, I'm coming . . . ."

SIGNS AND SYMPTOMS

- ☒ Involuntary sexual arousal
- ☒ Engorged labia, vulva, and clitoris
- ☒ Physical symptoms lasting for hours or even days
- ☒ Intense spontaneous orgasms
- ☒ Only short-term relief, or no relief at all, of arousal following orgasm

DIAGNOSIS AND TREATMENT

Treatment of PSAS/PGAD depends on what the suspected cause is.

- ☒ In cases where a nervous system disorder is suspected, treatments include nervous system and mood stabilizing medications such as Paxil, Prozac, Clonipin, and Zeprexa; topical anesthetics; surgical treatment of any lesions; and hormone normalization therapy.
- ☒ Anti-depressants—the side effect of decreased libido has helped some women
- ☒ Biofeedback
- ☒ Psychotherapy
- ☒ Electroshock therapy

PROGNOSIS

Management of PSAS/PGAD is challenging, but, with persistence, patients can get some control over the condition.

PREVALENCE

There are no accurate statistics as to the number of PSAS/PGAD cases.

HOW TO AVOID IT

There is no known way to avoid getting PSAS/PGAD.

NOTABLE CASES

No actual cases of PSAS/PGAD have risen to the level of fame, but the condition itself achieved a certain amount of notoriety when it was featured in the fifth season of the hit ABC TV show *Grey's Anatomy*. That was followed by actress Kristen Wiig's portrayal of a PSAS/PGAD sufferer on *Saturday Night Live* in October 2009—a send-up of the condition that angered many affected by it.

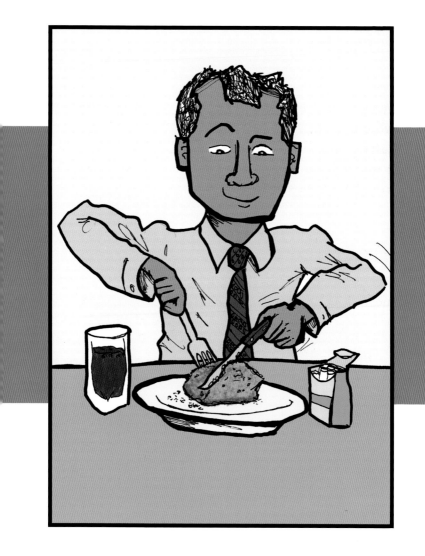

PICA

Imagine looking at a lightbulb and thinking, "Yum!" Or what if instead of popping open a can of Pringles to satisfy your hunger, you reached for a handful of dirt? It might sound nutty, but not for someone suffering from the rare disorder called pica.

WHAT IS IT?

Pica is an eating disorder in which sufferers ingest what medical researchers call "nonnutritive substances"—or what laypeople might call "stuff." What kind of stuff? Cigarette butts, sand, paint, stones, nails, lightbulbs, dirt, ash, wire, paper, clay, feces, pencils, erasers, plastic, chalk, wood, and coal all might be on the pica sufferer's menu. However, to the person with pica, eating these things doesn't seem odd at all.

The Upside of... Pica

- Never go hungry!
- Join the circus as the Amazing Lightbulb Eating Boy.
- Make cleanup time easy—just eat the mess.

Pica is most common in young children and adults with developmental disabilities, but has been seen in healthy adults as well.

ORIGINS

Pica is the Latin word for magpie, the notorious scavenger bird with a hearty—and indiscriminate—appetite.

WHAT CAUSES IT?

Nobody knows, although many theories abound. In practice, each case of pica must be evaluated on its own as to the causes. Some researchers believe it develops as a result of nutritional deficiencies. Other known factors that may contribute to the development of pica are parental neglect, developmental disorders, cultural factors, and psychological issues (e.g., anxiety, stress, or oral fixation).

Perhaps the most intriguing possible cause of pica is differing cultural attitudes toward what is and isn't acceptable to eat. So, for example, among pregnant African-American women, a commonly documented pica craving is for Argo laundry starch. The belief is that eating the laundry starch helps the baby's blood, and that it keeps the baby's skin smooth and clean. In writer Geri-Ann Galanti's 2004 book, *Caring for Patients from Different Cultures*, she writes that among African-American women, eating laundry starch is a carryover from the well-documented slave tradition of eating dirt or clay. In fact, ingesting dirt is a common practice throughout many non-Western areas of the world—and it even has an official scientific name, geophagy. According to Galanti, pregnant Mexican-

American women often crave magnesium carbonate (a form of chalk) or the ice that forms on the inside of the freezer. What's more, these women believe ignoring these cravings could cause birth defects or injuries to their unborn child.

SIGNS AND SYMPTOMS

Depending on the substance(s) being ingested, pica can either be harmless or deadly. Lead poisoning is a common consequence of pica, and other toxicity problems may arise depending on what's eaten. In addition, ingesting feces and dirt makes a patient vulnerable to any number of infectious and parasitic diseases. Other effects of pica include gastrointestinal issues such as constipation and bowel problems, and abrasions to the teeth from eating hard substances like rocks.

DIAGNOSIS AND TREATMENT

Because pica most often appears in children it can be difficult to diagnose. After all, to some extent we *expect* kids to eat disgusting stuff without a thought (one study says 25 to 30 percent of young kids eat stuff that normally isn't food). So in order for pica to be diagnosed, a person must regularly eat non-food items for a period lasting at least one month; and eating such items must be considered inappropriate for the person's developmental level. In terms of children, you'd expect a child to stop stuffing any old junk into his or her mouth at about eighteen to twenty-four months. Thus, the majority of cases are diagnosed in children aged two and three.

While children are the most likely pica sufferers, adults and adolescents are also afflicted. However, the overwhelming majority of adult cases occur in patients who are mentally retarded (in fact, pica is the most common eating disorder in mentally disabled adults). It is extremely rare in healthy adults.

Interestingly, another vulnerable population is pregnant women. While not common, in some women the usual oddball food cravings experienced during pregnancy are accompanied by a hunger for non-foodstuffs. According to the American Pregnancy Association, the most common items eaten by pregnant pica victims are dirt, clay, and laundry starch. Those three "delicacies" are followed in popularity by stones, burnt matches, charcoal, moth balls, ice, cornstarch, soap, sand, plaster, coffee grounds, baking soda, and cigarette ashes.

But no matter if pica appears in an adult or a child, when another mental disorder is present (e.g., schizophrenia, mental retardation, or severe developmental disabilities), pica is often hard to distinguish from the larger symptoms of those conditions. Thus, in such patients, treating pica will usually take a backseat to treating the more pervasive medical and psychological issues present.

Treatment of pica depends on the perceived causes of the disorder in a particular patient. If a nutritional deficiency is suspected, some patients have responded well once that deficiency is corrected. In most cases, a variety of behavioral therapies is successful in stopping or lessening the harmful effects of pica. In young children, pica often disappears on its own as the child develops.

PROGNOSIS

The prognosis for those with pica depends on what they eat. Obviously, if a person regularly ingests toxic materials, he or she might do lasting damage. In general, those with pica respond well to treatment and the condition is not harmful.

PREVALENCE

It's extraordinarily difficult to say how many people suffer from pica. It is without a doubt underreported, as well as underrecognized. Many parents no doubt just assume their child will outgrow eating inedible objects, or they may be too embarrassed to discuss such symptoms with their pediatrician.

HOW TO AVOID IT

There's no way to prevent pica. The best prevention right now is awareness. If you have young children, be aware of what they stick in their gobs.

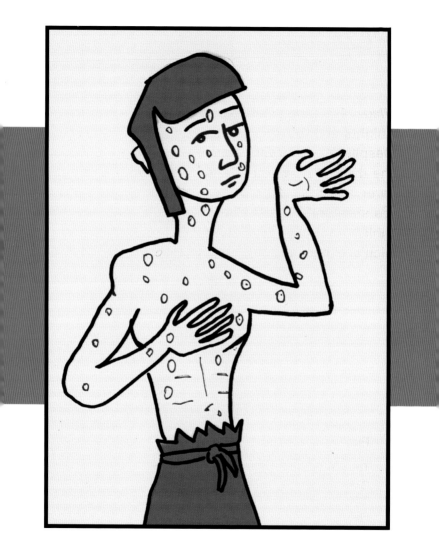

PLAGUE

Plague?!?! Didn't that go out around the same time as knights and jousts and wenches? Well, actually, no. Despite its medieval connotations, plague outlasted the days of King Arthur and Merlin. While it is much rarer today than at previous times in human history, it's still possible that you could come down with the biblical-sounding disease. And it ain't no mutton roast picnic, either.

The Upside of...
Plague

- The infectious disease that goes medieval on your ass.
- Gives the phrase, "Avoid it like the plague," a whole new meeting.
- Flea collars as the next hip accessory? You heard it here first.

WHAT IS IT?

Plague is a deadly infectious disease caused by the bacterium *Yersinia pesti*. There are actually three different forms of plague: bubonic, pneumonic, and septicemic (see "Signs and Symptoms," below, for more on each variety of plague).

ORIGINS

While no one knows exactly when plague first began, there are numerous references to the disease in art and written texts dating back to biblical times. What actually causes plague was a mystery until 1894, when two bacteriologists separately isolated the bacterium responsible. A vaccine was invented in 1896, and proved effective during an outbreak in India that year.

WHAT CAUSES IT?

Plague spreads through rodent populations when fleas infected with the *Yersinia pesti* bacterium pass it on as they dine on their rodent hosts. Humans contract plague by being bitten by an infected flea after coming into contact with an infected rodent or through exposure to rodent feces. It's also possible for plague to be transmitted between people if a person with pneumonic plague coughs or sneezes, and tiny infected droplets are breathed in by another person.

SIGNS AND SYMPTOMS

The signs and symptoms of plague depend on which of the three varieties of the disease one has.

▪ Bubonic Plague

Bubonic plague is the most common form of plague to affect humans. In bubonic plague the lymph glands are infected. (The term *bubonic* comes from the Greek word *bubo*, which means "swollen groin"—the groin, of course, being one site where lymph nodes reside).

People with bubonic plague will exhibit the following symptoms some two to five days after becoming infected:

- ☒ Pain in and swelling of the lymph glands—often in the groin, but also in the armpits or neck
- ☒ Flu-like symptoms: fever, muscle aches, headache, and chills

▪ Septicemic Plague

Septicemic plague occurs when the *Yersinia pesti* bacterium enters the bloodstream, usually through the lymphatic system or the respiratory system. Common symptoms include:

- ☒ Fever
- ☒ Abdominal pain
- ☒ Vomiting

- ☒ Chills
- ☒ Rapid heart rate
- ☒ Shock
- ☒ Blackened deadened skin—usually on the hands, feet, and nose—as a result of blood clots caused by toxins from the plague bacteria

- ■ **Pneumonic Plague**

Pneumonic plague is an infection of the lungs. It is transmitted through inhalation of infected respiratory droplets (e.g., when an infected person sneezes or coughs). Fortunately, pneumonic plague is the least prevalent form of the disease; unfortunately, it kills people quicker than either of the other two forms. The following symptoms of pneumonic plague typically show up two to four days after being infected, but may occur within hours.

- ☒ Headache
- ☒ Weakness
- ☒ Signs of pneumonia: coughing up blood, difficulty breathing, chest pain

DIAGNOSIS AND TREATMENT

A suspected diagnosis of plague can be confirmed by a blood test, analysis of saliva or respiratory discharge, or by taking a sample of lymphatic fluid.

The first thing to do if you suspect you have plague is to get to a hospital as quickly as you can and inform the medical staff. You must start treatment within twenty-four hours of the first appearance of symptoms.

Treatment consists first of isolating potential plague patients. Next you will receive antibiotics to combat the plague bacterium. The drugs will either be administered intravenously or into the muscles. A seven- to ten-day course of antibiotics is the norm. Depending on your condition, you also may be given oxygen, put on a ventilator, or given fluids intravenously.

PROGNOSIS

If left untreated, no matter what kind of plague you have, chances are damn good you're a goner. If treated quickly and effectively, the mortality rate from plague is less than 15 percent.

PREVALENCE

According to the World Health Organization there are 1,000 to 3,000 cases of plague every year. In the U.S., the Centers for Disease Control and Prevention says there are between ten and twenty cases a year. Today the disease is found mainly in semi-arid areas of Asia, Eastern Europe, Africa, South America, and North America. In the U.S., the largest number of cases has occurred in the desert Southwest.

HOW TO AVOID IT

Keep away from wild rodents, cats, and rabbits in known plague-infected areas.

NOTABLE CASES

As with influenza, plague outbreaks have been concentrated into a few major pandemics, as well as smaller flashes.

- **Plague of Justinian**

The Plague of Justinian is believed to have been the first plague pandemic. It occurred in 541 to 542 A.D., and struck the Byzantine Empire of Justinian I. The plague killed up to 5,000 people a day in the Byzantine capital of Constantinople. It went on to kill up to one quarter of the people living on the eastern side of the Mediterranean. Justinian I himself contracted the disease, but unlike so many under his rule he recovered.

- **Black Death**

The next, and most famous, outbreak of plague was the Black Death, which utterly devastated Europe from 1348 to 1350. There is some debate today as to whether the *Yersinia pesti* bacterium actually caused the Black Death, but it is still a widely held view. In any case, the death toll was staggering: estimates say between 30 and 60 percent of Europe's population died (25 to 50 million people), while worldwide up to 75 million people perished.

▪ Third Pandemic

For some reason, the third plague pandemic didn't get a catchy name. Nevertheless, it rivaled its predecessors in its destructiveness. The Third Pandemic began in China's Yunnan Province in 1855, and then spread to every continent of the globe. The hardest hit areas were China and India. Combined deaths in those two countries exceeded 12 million. Officially, the Third Pandemic lasted until 1959, when the World Health Organization said fewer than 200 plague cases were present worldwide.

▪ Los Angeles Plague of 1924

Hardly a pandemic, an outbreak of pneumonic plague in Los Angeles killed 37 people from late 1924 into early 1925. The L.A. flare-up was the last urban incidence of plague in the U.S.

▪ Plague as Biological Weapon

Along with other infectious diseases, such as anthrax and smallpox, plague is increasingly mentioned as a possible biological warfare agent. There is concern that an aerosolized version of the bacterium could be spread into the air by terrorists, causing an outbreak of pneumonic plague. Indeed, several reports indicate that during the Cold War, Soviet biological warfare specialists created just such a weapon.

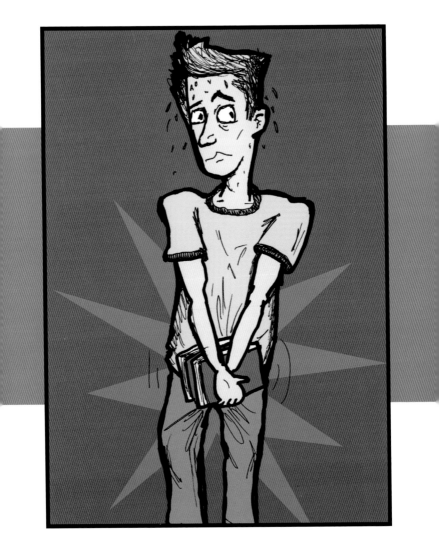

PRIAPISM

In these days of Viagra, men have a nice insurance policy against being unable to perform sexually. But what if instead of being unable to get it *up*, a man couldn't get it *down*? Talk about erectile dysfunction!

At first blush, having a rock-hard erection for hours might seem like a gift from God to some men. But this unfortunate scenario is actually a serious medical condition called priapism. If left untreated, priapism could result in permanent damage to the penis, making erections from sexual stimulation impossible.

WHAT IS IT?

Priapism is a disorder of the penis in which the patient experiences a prolonged unwanted erection. The erection occurs without sexual stimulation or arousal, and lasts for several hours, or sometimes even days.

ORIGINS

Priapism is named after Priapus, the Greek and Roman god of fertility. In ancient times, statues of Priapus featuring a giant erect phallus were placed in fields to ensure a good harvest.

WHAT CAUSES IT?

Before we discuss what goes wrong in priapism, let's first recall what we learned in sex ed, way back when. In a normal erection, physical or psychological arousal causes blood vessels in the soft tissue of the penis to expand and take in more blood. At the same time, other blood vessels in the penis constrict, so that the blood is trapped and the engorged penis stays erect. When the stimulation is over—ahem!—the constricted blood vessels relax, blood flows out of the penis, and it returns to its usual flaccid state. That's how things *normally* go.

In priapism, the system of blood flow to the penis breaks down somewhere, and the blood trapped in the erect Johnson just stays there. Blood flow to the penis is a complicated web of neurological and vascular functions, and it is extremely difficult to pinpoint just where the system is malfunctioning in cases of priapism. All that's known is that you're left with a painful swollen member.

To make matters a bit more complicated, there are two different varieties of priapism: ischemic priapism and nonischemic priapism, each with its own set of causes. *Ischemic* means there is a decrease in blood supply to an organ caused by constriction of blood vessels. Thus, in ischemic priapism, constricted blood vessels prevent blood from draining out of the penis, keeping it erect. This is the more common form of priapism, accounting for more than 95 percent of cases.

Ischemic priapism may be caused by:

- ☒ Blood disorders such as sickle cell disease and leukemia
- ☒ Prescription drugs such as erectile dysfunction drugs, blood pressure medication, antidepressants, and blood thinners
- ☒ Use of illicit drugs like marijuana, cocaine, and ecstasy—as well as recreational use of erectile dysfunction drugs
- ☒ Alcohol abuse
- ☒ Diabetes
- ☒ Spinal cord injury
- ☒ Anesthesia
- ☒ Bites from the Brazilian wandering spider

Nonischemic priapism, the less common form, occurs when the main artery in the penis ruptures, and thus too much blood continuously flows into the penis. Virtually all cases of nonischemic priapism result from trauma to the penis, genitals, pelvis, or perineum (the area between the penis and the anus).

SIGNS AND SYMPTOMS

Whether a case of priapism is ischemic or nonischemic, the one constant will be an erect penis that simply will not lie down. But there are different symptoms for each kind of priapism.

- **Symptoms of Ischemic Priapism**
  - ☒ PAIN!!!
  - ☒ The shaft of the penis will usually be hard and rigid, but the tip of the penis (known in medical terms as the glans) remains soft
  - ☒ Erection lasts from four hours up to several days if left untreated

- **Symptoms of Nonischemic Priapism**
  - ☒ Prolonged erection lasting up to four hours
  - ☒ Erect but not stiff penis
  - ☒ Little or no pain

DIAGNOSIS AND TREATMENT

A diagnosis of priapism is made when any other cause of prolonged erections is ruled out (such as Vegas call girls).

Needless to say, priapism should be treated as quickly as possible. If you, or someone you know, has an erection lasting four hours or more, swallow your pride and seek medical attention—fast! On the way to the doctor or the emergency room, an ice pack on your crotch may help relieve the pain of ischemic priapism. Once at the doc, the most common form of treatment is to aspirate the penis.

Aspiration means the doctor will put some local anesthetic on your Johnson, jab a syringe in your prick, and suck out the excess blood. This lovely process may be followed by the doc injecting saline solution into the penis's veins to flush them of the oxygen-poor blood. Sadly, one round of aspiration may not do the trick, and the process may have to be repeated several times until your member reaches flaccidity.

The Upside of...
Priapism

- Save money on Viagra.
- Impress your dates.
- Dread having to answer the question, "What's up?"

Another treatment is to inject the penis with medication that causes the blood vessels to relax and allow blood to flow out. The doctor may use drugs such as phenylephrine, epinephrine, norepinephrine, or metaraminol.

If the above methods fail, you may need surgery to implant a shunt. The shunt diverts blood flow and allows the blood to flow normally through the penis again.

In cases of nonischemic priapism, the erection often goes away on its own. Putting ice on the crotch or on the perineal area may alleviate the symptoms. In some cases, however, surgery may be required to repair damaged arteries and/or tissues, or to implant material that temporarily blocks blood flow to the penis and is then absorbed by the body. Again, it's best to see a doctor to discuss your options.

It's important to stress that priapism must be treated as quickly as possible. Left untreated, it could result in serious permanent damage to the penis. Over time, the blood trapped in the priapic penis becomes deoxygenated. This oxygen-poor blood is toxic to the penile tissues, and if it isn't drained, it will damage or destroy the tissues. Failure to treat priapism quickly can result in permanent impotence. The absolute worst case scenario in priapism is that gangrene sets in. If this unfortunate situation occurs, a patient may be looking at amputation of the penis as the only course of treatment!

PROGNOSIS

If treated in time, most patients with priapism are perfectly healthy and retain normal sexual function.

HOW TO AVOID IT

If the priapism is caused by a disease or other medical condition, treatment of the underlying condition should take care of the problem. Otherwise, try to avoid injuries to the penis, and take it easy on the drugs and alcohol.

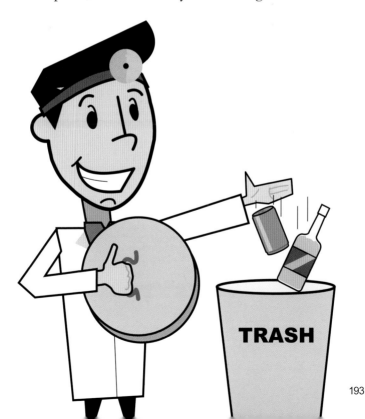

TRASH

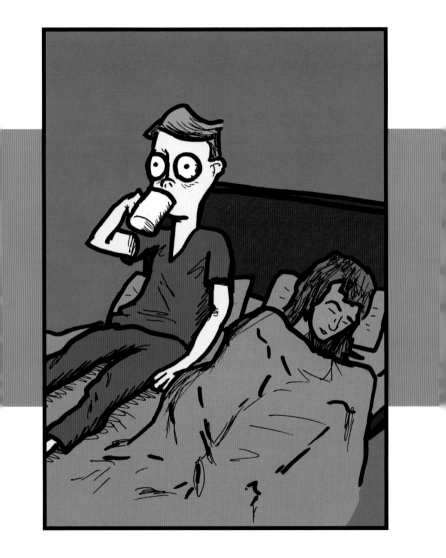

PRIMARY ALVEOLAR HYPOVENTILATION, CONGENITAL CENTRAL HYPOVENTILATION SYNDROME (CCHS), ONDINE'S CURSE

Ah, sleep. Sweet, blissful sleep. Is there anything better than sinking into your bed when you're completely drained and drifting off to dreamland? Well, what if you lived in fear of falling asleep, because the simple act of slipping into unconsciousness was enough to kill you? That's exactly the fear that people suffering from primary alveolar hypoventilation must deal with every day.

WHAT IS IT?

Primary alveolar hypoventilation or congenital central hypoventilation syndrome (CCHS) is a respiratory disorder in which people stop breathing during sleep. It is a rare and potentially deadly form of sleep apnea, a rather common condition wherein breathing is interrupted during sleep. But in CCHS, the central nervous system function that keeps us breathing while we're unconscious (called autonomic breathing) is damaged.

ORIGINS

The popular term Ondine's curse comes from a German folktale. Ondine was a water nymph who married a human and gave birth to his child, thus giving up her immortality for love. At their wedding her husband declared, "My every waking breath shall be my pledge of love and faithfulness to you." When Ondine later discovered her husband's unfaithfulness, she placed a curse on him: echoing his vow at their wedding, she told him he'd be able to breathe when he was awake, but should he fall asleep his breathing would stop and he would die. Although he tried to remain awake, eventually the husband drifted off to sleep, and per the curse, his breathing halted and he perished.

The disorder was first described in 1962 by two researchers studying apnea.

WHAT CAUSES IT?

In the majority of cases, CCHS is present at birth. In patients with congenital CCHS, a gene mutation of the PHOX2B gene is the suspected cause. Other, rarer, causes are traumatic brain injury, stroke, or a complication of neurosurgery.

SIGNS AND SYMPTOMS

- ☒ Death
- ☒ Night apnea
- ☒ Difficulty breathing or total loss of breathing
- ☒ Abnormal pupils
- ☒ Gastroesophageal reflux disease (GERD)
- ☒ Seizures
- ☒ Fainting
- ☒ Pneumonia

DIAGNOSIS AND TREATMENT

The first step in diagnosing Ondine's curse is to rule out other issues that could affect breathing, such as muscular dystrophy or emphysema. A chest x-ray may be performed, as well as tests of pulmonary function and evaluation of the patient's neurological function.

Treatments for Ondine's curse vary. In some patients medication that stimulates respiratory function helps. A mechanical ventilator is required anytime the patient sleeps.

PROGNOSIS

Many children born with CCHS do not survive infancy. Any respiratory infection is enough to overwhelm their fragile systems. But as children grow and become stronger, they have a better chance of survival. Some 65 percent of CCHS patients are able to breathe during the day without mechanical help (although all patients need a ventilator at night).

PREVALENCE

Ondine's curse affects about 1 in 200,000 newborns.

HOW TO AVOID IT

As with any condition caused by a genetic mutation, there's not much you can do to prevent it.

The Upside of...
CCHS

- Convenient excuse to stay out all night.
- Well, there goes sleeping on the job . . .
- Break Guinness World Record for counting sheep.
